© Dr Christopher B Maclay 2024

METFORMIN

Preventing Diabetes and Chronic Disease

Dr Christopher B. Maclay

Kindle Direct Publishing, 2024

© Dr. Christopher Maclay 2024

Copyright © 2024 by Dr. Christopher B. Maclay
All rights Reserved.
No part of this publication may be reproduced, distributed or transmitted in any form or by any means, including photocopying, recording, or other electronic or mechanical methods, without the prior written permission of the publisher, except as permitted by copyright law. For permission requests, contact the author via his webpage:
www.maclaymedical.com.au

Book Cover by Dr. Christopher B. Maclay
Independently published with Kindle Direct Publishing
Language English
ISBN: 9798342648288
1 Edition 2024

Important Notice to Readers
The information provided in this book is for educational and informational purposes only. It is not medical advice. The content represents the personal views and opinions of the author. It is not intended to replace consultation with a qualified healthcare provider. Readers are encouraged to seek personal medical advice from their healthcare professionals before implementing any treatment, supplement or protocol discussed in this book, especially those involving dietary, lifestyle, or medical interventions for ageing and age-related diseases.

While every effort has been made to ensure that the information provided is accurate and up to date at the time of publication, medical knowledge and research in the field of functional, anti-aging and regenerative medical therapy, preventative health and pharmacotherapy is constantly evolving. The author and publisher do not accept any liability for inaccuracies or omissions, nor for any potential adverse effects or outcomes resulting from the application of information presented in this book.

Always consult with a licensed healthcare provider before making decisions about your health.

About the Author

Dr. Christopher Maclay, MBBS, FRACGP is a Medical Doctor, Author, Health Writer, Blogger and Health Coach. Dr Maclay has a persisting interest in Functional, Anti-Ageing and Regenerative Medicine (FAARM). Dr. Maclay lived and studied in Argentina in South America, after which he returned to his hometown of Melbourne, Australia where he undertook Residency and Fellowship training.

His interest in unorthodox approaches to medicine began in 2012 upon completion of training with ACNEM, (the Australian College of Nutritional and Environmental Medicine). He has also trained with A4M (American Anti-Ageing Association of Medicine), Bio balance (Walsh Research Institute) and worked briefly in Chronic Fatigue Research at Griffiths University, in Queensland, Australia. He is or has been a member of ACNEM, AIMA (Australian Integrative Medicine Association), RACGP Integrative Medicine Special Interests, IPS (International Peptide Society), A4M (The American Academy of Anti Aging Medicine).

In 2024 Dr Maclay indulged his passion for writing, investigating and advocacy in the world of FAARM with the first book in this series 'Stop Ageing'. With 20 years of experience, he is contactable via his website.

www.maclaymedical.com.au

METFORMIN

TABLE OF CONTENTS

Forward — 9

Introduction — 11

Chapter 1: The Global Health Crisis – Why We Need Preventative Health Now — 16
   WHAT WOULD WE LOOK FOR IN A PREVENTATIVE HEALTH INTERVENTION IN THE FACE OF THIS WAVE OF CHRONIC DISEASE? — 29

Chapter 2: The Current Approach to Preventative Health – Where Are We Now? — 34
   The RACGP Red Book — 43

Chapter 3: Metformin – A Drug for the Masses — 50

Chapter 5: Metformin in Diabetes Prevention — 67

Chapter 6: Metformin and Prevention of Cardiovascular Disease — 78

Chapter 7: Metformin and Cancer Prevention — 85

© Dr. Christopher Maclay 2024

Chapter 8: Metformin and Chronic Kidney Disease Prevention	94
Chapter 9: Metformin and Prevention of Dementia Syndromes.	102
Chapter 10: Estimating healthspan and lifespan extension from the preventative use of metformin.	108
Chapter 10: How will Industry react?	114
Chapter 11: A Comprehensive Risk-Benefit Analysis	121
Chapter 12: The TAME Trial	128
Chapter 13: Beyond Metformin – The Future of Preventative Health	132
Conclusion	139
EXTRAS	142
Thought Leaders	143
Further Reading	145

METFORMIN

'A preventative intervention in time saves nine.'

Or...

'A preventative intervention in the hand is worth two in the bush.'

Or more simply...

'A preventative intervention a day, keeps Big Pharma away.'

Forward

The world is in desperate need of safe and effective interventions to prevent chronic disease. Metformin, a cheap, effective, and safe medicine with decades of use, may well be the most under-utilised tool in the fight against chronic disease. In 'Metformin: Prevent Diabetes and Chronic Disease.', Dr. Christopher Maclay explores how this widely prescribed drug has the potential to address many of the root metabolic dysfunctions driving some of the most important of the so-called 'age and lifestyle' related illnesses.

Current preventative health strategies are failing to prevent the overwhelming growth in chronic diseases like Diabetes, Chronic Kidney Disease, Cardiovascular disease, Cancer, and Dementia. They focus largely on vaccination, early detection and lifestyle advice. Priority is given to expensive and poorly effective 'management of chronic disease'. Dr. Maclay argues for a shift toward targeting the underlying metabolic processes that contribute to these conditions, with metformin leading the charge.

Backed by an abundance of clinical data, metformin has proven efficacy in preventing multiple chronic diseases, underscoring the immediate need to repurpose existing therapies like metformin to mitigate the growing public health crisis.

Many in our community are realising that there is no 'centralised plan' to keep them well. This growing body of informed individuals seeking life prolonging and improving interventions will find 'Metformin' an up-to-date review of Metformin's role in both personalised and mass preventative health interventions.

© Dr. Christopher Maclay 2024

METFORMIN

Introduction

Metformin has been available for decades. It has been used by millions of people worldwide. Its mechanism of action and safety profile are well known. Furthermore, it is cheap, and off patent. Metformin has been shown in trial after trial to mitigate the risk of developing Obesity, Metabolic Dysfunction, Diabetes, Cardiovascular Disease, Chronic Kidney Disease and Cancer. The diagnosis of these very diseases is exploding in numbers, constituting a true worldwide pandemic of Chronic Disease. These and other factors made Meformin an ideal candidate for wide scale preventative health applications. What is impeding the more widespread use of metformin?

Metformin has been a staple in the treatment of type 2 diabetes for over six decades, offering millions of people a reliable, safe, and effective means of managing their blood sugar levels. With a long-established history, it has proven itself to be not only one of the most widely used medications globally but also one of the most affordable, safe and accessible. For many, it remains a lifeline against the complications of diabetes, improving both quality of life and long-term health outcomes. But what if its potential reaches far beyond diabetes management?

Over the years, an increasing body of research has begun to unveil a broader, more powerful role for metformin. Its unique mechanisms of action, targeting insulin sensitivity and reducing hepatic glucose production, actions in the mitochondria and effects on lipid profiles and inflammation, have profound implications for a range of conditions that plague modern society—conditions such as obesity, metabolic syndrome, cardiovascular disease, and even cancer. These chronic diseases, often intertwined with lifestyle factors and the global rise of obesity, represent an enormous public health burden, driving morbidity, mortality, and escalating healthcare costs.

Metformin, however, has emerged as a candidate capable of addressing many of these conditions at their root. Its ability to regulate metabolic pathways, reduce systemic inflammation, and promote longevity at the cellular level has drawn attention from researchers and clinicians alike. Numerous trials have consistently shown that metformin reduces the risk of cardiovascular events, improves metabolic function, and may even inhibit cancer onset and progression. These promising outcomes have fuelled interest in using metformin not only as a treatment but as a preventative tool—a medication that could be used to forestall the onset of chronic diseases in high-risk populations.

Metformin has a very favourable and well-known safety profile, beyond the clinical benefits adding to its appeal. For a drug that has been used by millions worldwide, the rates of significant side effects are remarkably low. In most cases, metformin is well tolerated, with gastrointestinal discomfort being the most common issue—an issue that often resolves with time or dose adjustment. Its affordability, with generic versions available globally, adds another layer to its suitability for large-scale use in preventative health. At a time when the costs of treating chronic diseases continue to skyrocket, metformin offers an inexpensive alternative that could reduce the economic strain on healthcare systems. An option available to both poor and rich countries alike.

So, why hasn't metformin been more widely adopted as a preventative medication? If it is cheap, safe, and effective, why isn't it prescribed more broadly for conditions like obesity, cardiovascular disease, and even cancer? The answer lies in a complex interplay of factors.

First, there is the entrenched focus of modern medicine on treating or 'managing' disease rather than preventing it. Preventative health, while increasingly acknowledged as essential, has yet to take its rightful place in mainstream medical practice. Metformin, as a preventative tool, represents a shift in thinking—a proactive approach that challenges the reactive nature of much of healthcare today.

Additionally, regulatory hurdles and the lack of widespread professional and public awareness limit metformin's use outside of diabetes. Despite the wealth of research supporting its benefits for non-diabetic conditions, official guidelines have been slow to reflect these findings. The gap between scientific evidence and clinical practice is often wide, and in the case of metformin, it has left many potential beneficiaries without access to this life-changing medication. Concerns about over-prescription, especially in healthy individuals, also linger, even though the risks associated with metformin are minimal compared to the risks posed by the chronic diseases it can delay and prevent.

Moreover, pharmaceutical and healthcare industries face their own challenges when it comes to advocating for metformin. Unlike newer, patent-protected drugs, metformin offers little financial incentive for promotion. Which pharmaceutical giant would sponsor such a trial? As a generic medication, it lacks the commercial backing that typically drives new treatments to the forefront of clinical practice. This has resulted in less advocacy for its expanded use, despite the overwhelming evidence of its benefits.

This book, third in a series about Functional, Anti-Ageing and Regenerative Medicine, seeks to uncover the untapped potential of metformin as a preventative health intervention. We will explore its role in mitigating the risks of chronic diseases that dominate modern life—obesity, metabolic dysfunction, cardiovascular disease, and cancer—and delve into the mechanisms that make it such a powerful tool. We will also examine the barriers preventing its widespread adoption and discuss how these can be overcome to transform the way we approach chronic disease prevention.

By highlighting the scientific research, clinical trials, and real-world evidence behind metformin, this book aims to provide a comprehensive understanding of why this humble medication could hold the key to a healthier future – partly through its own pharmacological profile and partly through popularising true preventative health interventions. The time has come to rethink our approach to chronic disease, shifting from costly treatments to affordable prevention. In a world where metabolic dysfunction is rampant and the burden of chronic disease continues to rise, metformin offers a beacon of hope—a simple, well-tolerated, and affordable intervention with the potential to change lives.

There is really no question that metformin works. The question is simply, what are we waiting for to prioritise preventative health interventions? Recognising Metformin as an ideal candidate can set a precedent allowing clinicians and patients to finally target prevention specifically.

METFORMIN

Chapter 1: The Global Health Crisis – Why We Need Preventative Health Now

The Surging Tide of Chronic Disease

The world faces an unprecedented rise in the incidence and prevalence of Chronic Diseases, which now stand as the leading cause of death and disability worldwide. These diseases—cancer, cardiovascular disease, dementia, diabetes, chronic kidney disease and other metabolic disorders—are not just numbers and statistics. These are real people, mothers, fathers, sisters and brothers. They represent real suffering, lives cut short and immeasurable human loss. It is estimated that Chronic Diseases now account for 71% of all deaths globally, with cardiovascular disease alone responsible for 17.9 million deaths each year, followed closely by cancer and respiratory diseases. Horrific. But what if we can prevent these illnesses? Would you, as I do, feel a sense of urgency to do so?

By way of example Type 2 Diabetes, once rare, has become a modern epidemic, with an estimated 537 million adults living with the condition as of 2021. This number is projected to rise to 643 million by 2030. At the same time, neurodegenerative diseases like Alzheimer's and other dementias are growing rapidly, particularly in ageing populations, threatening to overburden healthcare systems worldwide. Again, the statistics are slightly numbing. 55 MILLION individuals living with dementia now, some 78 million by 2030.

These illnesses are not random events, they share strong, measurable, well understood and common metabolic dysfunctions at their source. Metabolic dysfunctions that can be treated. Many of these diseases are indeed 'lifestyle related'. But what does that mean? Why is 'lifestyle related' given as an excuse to avoid preventative treatment? How many times have we heard association does not prove causality?

'Lifestyle related' means the current social, political, cultural environment we exist in is associated with the disease promoting behaviours we humans exhibit in these environments.

It also means that efforts to alter the environment to encourage other less 'pathogenic' behaviours is possible.

It does NOT mean humans are making decision to get sick. It does not attribute blame. It is not an excuse not to treat preventatively.

We would have to be blind not to notice the financial interests of agricultural, food manufacturing, pharmaceutical giants, banks and construction companies have become deeply embedded in the legislative and regulatory framework of our societies. Through there lobbying, marketing, influence on popular culture, professional education, regulation and the development of guidelines are intimately responsible for the creation of this disease promoting environment. Intentionally or otherwise.

When those responsible for the disease promoting characteristics of our modern environment feel their interests are served by promoting change – change tends to occur. The inverse is also true. When change opposes the interests of 'industry' it does not. Adding insult to injury there is a sometimes implicit and often explicit accusation that 'poor lifestyle' is the fault of the population – as if these changes happened isolation. As if wrenching children out of their homes from a young age doesn't change their eating habits. As if the food pyramids are unbiased. As if baby formula is a substitute for mother's milk. As if fast food chains sold food, and not food like products. As if approving the sale of phones and 'iPads' with no effective warnings or controls on the harm they cause is unrelated and not worthy of conversation. They charge the public to live in this new ecosystem, accept no liability for the side effects and attribute moral blame to them for living in it.

Furthermore, to state that lifestyle is the cause of the Chronic Disease epidemic would be misleading – by far the biggest 'risk factor' for chronic disease is age. No matter how little exercise or how poorly a 15-year-old eats they will not get dementia. Biological age, the state of your cells, tissues and organs, is the biggest driver of chronic disease. Sedentary lifestyles, poor dietary intake, and exploding rates of obesity and metabolic dysfunction are, unsurprisingly, accelerating the rise of these conditions.

Chronic Diseases are not just a medical problem, they are a societal and civilisational one. Without a shift in approach, this rising tide will only swell, leaving individuals, families, and already ill-equipped health systems overwhelmed and unable to cope.
Accelerated by modern diets and lifestyles that are by design or otherwise deficient in what we need and overloaded in what we do not. Too little outdoor activity, too little vitamin d, magnesium, soluble fibre. Too little social interaction, sleep. Too much screen time, sugar, sedentarism. Too much artificial light.

In this kind of modern environment – asking people to change their diet and lifestyle - has had quite predictable outcomes. Few. The Chronic Disease burden continues to rise alarmingly.

Having said this, many of these metabolic changes are preventable (cheap) and treatable (expensive). In this context expensive could be substituted for the word 'profitable'.

The Cost of Treating Chronic Illness

The economic burden of treating chronic diseases is staggering. As lifespans increase and more people live longer with these conditions, healthcare costs are soaring. In the United States alone, the cost of chronic diseases is estimated to reach $4.2 trillion annually by 2030, accounting for 80% of the total healthcare expenditure. How much is spent on prevention? And of the expenditure ear marked for 'prevention', how much actually avoids the development of chronic illness? Europe and many other developing nations are witnessing similar trends.

For individuals, these costs manifest as lifelong medical bills, lost productivity, and personal financial ruin. The expenses tied to cancer treatments, diabetes management, cardiovascular surgeries, and long-term care for neurodegenerative diseases like dementia are unsustainable for most households. Many people are left to choose between life-saving treatments and financial security.

From a societal perspective, the costs of chronic disease ripple far beyond healthcare budgets. Lost productivity from sick days, disability, and early death reduces workforce participation, which impacts national economies and hampers growth. Governments are forced to allocate increasing amounts of public funds to care for those with preventable illnesses, which siphons resources from other pressing needs like education, infrastructure, and economic development. Prevention is always the cheaper option.

The question we are forced to confront is whether it is possible to turn the tide—to reduce these enormous costs by preventing these diseases from developing in the first place.

Mortality and Morbidity: The Human Toll

Chronic diseases are not just about financial burden—they profoundly impact quality of life. Unlike infectious diseases, which tend to strike quickly and resolutely, chronic diseases often develop over many years, leading to prolonged suffering and disability. Chronic disease is the true ageing or organs and systems, and without treatment and even with standard medical treatment they rarely resolve but are instead 'managed' to avoid worse consequences. Cardiovascular disease, for example, can result in heart attacks, strokes, and heart failure, leaving survivors with lasting physical limitations and reduced quality of life. Receiving a diagnosis of a Chronic Disease with the implication of lifelong management is an enormous stress in the life of an individual.

Dementia robs individuals of their memories, independence, and identity, while placing an overwhelming weight on caregivers. Diabetes, left unmanaged, can lead to amputations, kidney failure, and blindness, contributing to a cycle of physical and emotional suffering.

At the core of the issue is that chronic disease affects not only longevity (lifespan) but the quality of the years lived (healthspan). It's not just about how long we live, but how well we live. As people age, they deserve to maintain their independence, remain active, and enjoy life, but chronic disease strips them of these opportunities. Many of these diseases are progressive and incurable, and once diagnosed, they require lifelong management. With the growing number of people developing these conditions, the question we must ask is: **How much longer can we afford to treat, rather than prevent?**

Missed Opportunities in Prevention

One of the greatest failings of modern healthcare systems is their overwhelming focus on treatment rather than prevention. Across the globe, healthcare spending disproportionately favours addressing disease once it has already occurred, rather than investing in strategies that could prevent it altogether. This is unusual in human activity – there is a culture wide acceptance that prevention is better than cure, and in the case of health this is most certainly the case. Many suspect this is motivated more by financial interests, specifically the lucrative market of 'managing disease'. This reactive model dominates healthcare, particularly in developed nations, where the focus is on acute care, pharmaceutical interventions, and costly medical procedures. Where prevention is possible, emphasis is pushed towards early detection (not truly prevention) or 'lifestyle change' which while noble, is hardly concordant with the nature or severity of the disease process and is not slowing the rise in diagnosis. The concept of Chronic Disease Management is pervasive. Society has been educated to accept that Chronic Diseases cannot be cured, (or maybe even prevented?) and must instead by managed.

Science disagrees. We have known for decades that many chronic diseases are preventable. Research has consistently shown that simple lifestyle changes—diet, increasing physical activity, weight, stress, tobacco and alcohol use—can dramatically reduce the risk of developing most chronic diseases. What about medical interventions? If you are diagnosed with pneumonia, we don't recommend more walking and less sugar. We treat the illness. Why not approach preventative health like this?

METFORMIN

In the long, asymptomatic lead up to the diagnosis of a chronic disease medicine has years to intervene. Yet, public health systems and governments have procrastinated in the implementation of effective prevention programs at a large scale. And why wouldn't they, when the research efforts, systems in place to review and promote evidence and compilation of clinical practice guidelines are largely dominated by the financial interests of industry. To say otherwise is simply to avoid seeing the truth. I don't think anyone seriously challenges this assertion.

Barriers to prevention are multifaceted. On a policy level, is there insufficient funding and/or political will to shift resources toward prevention efforts? On an individual level, lifestyle changes are difficult to sustain without comprehensive support, and the social and environmental factors that drive unhealthy behaviours—such as poverty, lack of access to nutritious foods, sedentary workplaces and most of modern society — are pervasive; characteristics that are difficult for individuals to overcome. Furthermore, preventive health often lacks the immediacy that treatment demands, and as a result, receives less attention and fewer resources. Perhaps the public health czars could better justify their existence by guiding the research and policy in this direction? Is this too much to ask?

Additionally, there is the issue of health literacy. Many individuals are simply unaware of how their everyday choices affect their long-term health. Educational initiatives are needed to empower people to take control of their health and make informed decisions about diet, exercise, and other lifestyle factors. Regulatory efforts at arm's length from industry to ensure access to healthy spaces, foods, drinks which are biologically appropriate for humans not just profitable to produce and sell.

Beyond the diet and lifestyle interventions, there is an enormous void in TREATING PREVENTATIVELY. We don't tell people with a fracture to get more exercise and drink less alcohol, we treat them. In the same way, can't osteoporosis be avoided by ensuring Vitamin D and K2 supplementation as we did with rickets. Is it a coincidence that Rickets is not expensive (read profitable) to manage while osteoporosis is? We use statins to prevent cardiovascular disease, why not use metformin to prevent diabetes rather than waiting for it to be established? This medical prevention is an enormous chapter waiting to be written – and to date largely ignored by the Acute Allopathic Medicine Model and its guidelines. They see people as well one day and sick the next, with no interventions in the intervening pre-clinical phase – the phase which is perfect for effective, low cost and low risk interventions. Right the ship *before* the sails are in the water.

The reality is that the global health crisis we now face is largely preventable. Yet, without a significant shift toward prevention, the situation will only worsen. Our best bet is finding an alignment of interests between protecting public finances, patient well-being and public opinion.

The Time for Change: A Preventive Health Revolution

The need for a revolution in how we approach healthcare has never been more urgent. The current model, focused on treating disease after it has manifested, is unsustainable both economically and socially. It is time for a paradigm shift—a move toward preventative health on a wide scale, where the focus is on stopping disease before it starts.

Preventative health is not a new concept, but its importance has been greatly under-appreciated. The idea of investing in health upfront to avoid the development of disease is both logical and cost-effective. It is far cheaper to prevent a heart attack than to treat one. It is far more humane to stop the progression of Alzheimer's before it begins than to manage the advanced stages of the disease.

In what seems a relatively bizarre twist of fate Metformin, the topic of this book, offers a unique opportunity in this regard. It should be a boring drug. But with its proven safety, affordability, and ability to prevent or mitigate many chronic diseases, it could serve as a cornerstone in the broader application of preventative health. Furthermore, I think it will open the flood gates for further re purposing and of existing treatments (and development of new ones) targeting the pathological metabolism causing chronic disease. Metformin alone cannot change the healthcare landscape. What is needed is a concerted effort to prioritise prevention at every level—from individual behaviour changes to systemic health policy reform. I for one am tired of waiting for a top-down change.

The time for action is now. Governments, healthcare providers, and individuals must embrace a new vision for health—one that sees prevention as the key to a healthier, longer, and more sustainable future. The costs of inaction are too great, and the benefits of prevention are too significant to ignore.

Diagnosing more people with Chronic Diseases and at Younger Ages

Chronic diseases such as cardiovascular disease, diabetes, cancer, and neurodegenerative disorders are not only increasing in prevalence but are also being diagnosed at progressively younger ages. The burden of these diseases, which have historically been associated with aging populations, is shifting towards younger demographics due to various lifestyle, environmental, and socio-economic factors. This trend has significant implications for public health systems and underscores the urgent need for effective preventive strategies.

Obesity, which is a significant risk factor for multiple chronic diseases, has become an epidemic in its own right, with over 650 million adults worldwide classified as obese in 2016 (WHO, 2016). This epidemic has had a profound impact on the earlier onset of chronic conditions like type 2 diabetes, cardiovascular disease, and even certain cancers.

Cancer, another traditionally age-related condition, is also being diagnosed earlier. The incidence of colorectal cancer, for instance, has been rising among younger adults. Research published in the Journal of the National Cancer Institute found that the incidence of colorectal cancer in adults under 50 years of age increased by 2% annually between 1998 and 2013 (Siegel et al., 2017). The exact reasons for this rise are unclear, but researchers point to diet, obesity, and environmental factors as potential contributors.

Additionally, neurodegenerative diseases, such as Alzheimer's disease, are increasingly being identified in middle-aged adults. While most cases are still diagnosed in older individuals, early-onset Alzheimer's (diagnosed before age 65) is becoming more common, with an estimated 5-6% of all Alzheimer's cases falling into this category (Alzheimer's Association, 2021).

More diagnosis, less cures, more people under management.

The prevalence of chronic diseases has been rising globally, particularly in high-income countries, but is also becoming a major issue in low- and middle-income nations. According to the World Health Organization (WHO), chronic diseases account for 71% of all deaths globally, with cardiovascular diseases leading the charge, followed by cancers, respiratory diseases, and diabetes (WHO, 2021). The burden of chronic diseases is expected to grow as populations age, but the accelerated pace of these diseases appearing earlier in life is contributing to a widespread public health crisis.

For example, diabetes has seen a sharp increase in prevalence, particularly among younger adults. The International Diabetes Federation reports that the number of people aged 20-79 living with diabetes increased from 151 million in 2000 to 463 million in 2019 and is projected to rise to 700 million by 2045 (IDF Diabetes Atlas, 2019). A growing number of these cases are being diagnosed in people in their 30s and 40s, driven largely by rising rates of obesity and sedentary lifestyles.

Similarly, cardiovascular disease (CVD), once predominantly diagnosed in older adults, is increasingly being identified in younger populations. A study from the American Heart Association found that between 1995 and 2014, the prevalence of heart attacks among people aged 35-54 increased, particularly among women (Wilmot et al., 2015). This trend is fuelled by risk factors such as obesity, hypertension, and diabetes, which are also on the rise in younger individuals.

Implications for Public Health

The rising prevalence and earlier onset of chronic diseases present significant challenges for public health systems worldwide. Younger populations are not only developing chronic diseases earlier, but they are also experiencing these diseases for a longer portion of their lives, leading to increased healthcare costs, greater disability, and reduced quality of life. This trend further underscores the importance of implementing effective preventive interventions, such as promoting healthy lifestyles and considering pharmacological approaches like metformin, which has shown promise in delaying the onset of multiple chronic conditions (Barzilai et al., 2016).

Without swift and comprehensive action to address the root causes of this trend, the global burden of chronic disease is set to continue increasing, placing unprecedented strain on healthcare systems and economies worldwide.

References

1. World Health Organization. (2021). Noncommunicable diseases. Retrieved from https://www.who.int/news-room/fact-sheets/detail/noncommunicable-diseases
2. International Diabetes Federation. (2019). IDF Diabetes Atlas (9th ed.). Retrieved from https://diabetesatlas.org/
3. Wilmot, K. A., et al. (2015). Sex differences in coronary heart disease risk factors: Insights from the Framingham Heart Study. Journal of the American Heart Association, 4(7), e001768.
4. World Health Organization. (2016). Obesity and overweight. Retrieved from https://www.who.int/news-room/fact-sheets/detail/obesity-and-overweight
5. Siegel, R. L., et al. (2017). Colorectal cancer incidence patterns in the United States, 1974–2013. *Journal of the National Cancer Institute*, 109(8), djx073.
6. Alzheimer's Association. (2021). Alzheimer's disease facts and figures. Retrieved from https://www.alz.org/alzheimers-dementia/facts-figures
7. Barzilai, N., et al. (2016). Metformin as a tool to target aging. Cell Metabolism 23(6), 1060-1065.

METFORMIN

WHAT WOULD WE LOOK FOR IN A PREVENTATIVE HEALTH INTERVENTION IN THE FACE OF THIS WAVE OF CHRONIC DISEASE?

Characteristics of a Perfect Preventive Health Intervention

The concept of an ideal preventive health intervention has been widely explored in medical literature, particularly as healthcare systems shift their focus from treatment to prevention. A perfect preventive health intervention would aim to reduce the burden of disease, promote long-term health, have minimal risks and be cost effective. While no intervention may be perfect in practice, there are key characteristics that can define an optimal preventive strategy. Below are the essential features of such an intervention, backed by research and expert analysis.

1. Efficacy in Preventing Multiple Diseases
An ideal preventive intervention would target the biological mechanisms that contribute to a broad range of chronic diseases, thereby reducing the incidence of conditions like cardiovascular disease, diabetes, cancer, neurodegenerative diseases, and others. This multifaceted approach is crucial, as many chronic diseases share common risk factors, including inflammation, insulin resistance, and metabolic dysfunction.

Metformin works by addressing metabolic pathways common to conditions such as diabetes, cardiovascular disease, chronic kidney disease, dementia and even some cancers (Barzilai et al., 2016). Preventive interventions that can address root causes across various diseases are more effective and efficient for public health.

2. Safety and Minimal Side Effects

A key criterion for a successful preventive intervention is its safety profile, particularly for long-term use in otherwise healthy individuals. The risks of the intervention should be minimal, and side effects should be mild and manageable. Long term data is always preferable. This is especially important for interventions aimed at the general population, as the risks must not outweigh the benefits.

Metformin, for example, has a well-documented safety profile with decades of clinical use, making it a strong candidate for preventive applications. Although it carries minor risks, such as gastrointestinal upset or rare cases of lactic acidosis (calculated at 1 in 30,000) in individuals with renal impairment, its risk-benefit ratio is generally favourable for high-risk populations (Inzucchi et al., 2014).

3. Affordability and Accessibility

An ideal preventive intervention must be affordable and widely accessible to the general population. Cost-effectiveness is a critical consideration, especially for large-scale public health initiatives, as expensive interventions can widen health disparities. In this context, generic drugs like metformin are often highlighted for their affordability compared to newer medications, making them viable options for widespread preventive use (Pollak, 2012).

Moreover, the perfect intervention should be easy to distribute, allowing for rapid and efficient scaling across diverse populations and healthcare settings. The use of affordable interventions has been shown to dramatically reduce the incidence of preventable diseases, as seen in large-scale vaccination programs and preventive cardiovascular treatments (Murray et al., 2012).

4. Evidence-Based and Supported by Strong Clinical Data

For a preventive intervention to be widely adopted, it must be grounded in robust, evidence-based research. This includes well-designed clinical trials, long-term studies, and a clear understanding of the biological mechanisms involved. Ideally, the intervention would have demonstrated efficacy in both preventing disease and extending healthspan.

Metformin is currently undergoing extensive research in trials like the TAME (Targeting Aging with Metformin) trial, which aims to demonstrate its role in delaying aging and preventing multiple age-related diseases (Barzilai et al., 2016). We will discuss the TAME trial specifically later.

5. Feasibility for Implementation and Monitoring

The ease of implementing and monitoring the intervention is another key factor. A perfect preventive intervention would be easy to administer, requiring minimal specialized equipment or expertise, and it would allow for straightforward monitoring of outcomes. This aspect is particularly important for public health interventions that need to be delivered to large populations.

Additionally, it is important that the intervention does not require constant medical supervision or invasive procedures, thus ensuring compliance and minimizing the burden on healthcare systems. Metformin, for example, is an oral medication that is relatively easy to monitor with regular blood tests and does not require complex medical infrastructure for its administration.

6. Capacity for Personalization

An ideal preventive intervention would also allow for personalization, catering to individual risk factors, genetic predispositions, and personal health profiles. Personalized preventive medicine can optimize outcomes by tailoring interventions to those who stand to benefit the most while minimizing unnecessary treatment for low-risk individuals (Collins & Varmus, 2015).

In personalized healthcare models, interventions like metformin can be selectively used in individuals with risk factors for chronic diseases, such as obesity, metabolic syndrome, or a strong family history of chronic illnesses, enhancing its preventive impact while reducing exposure to unnecessary risk.

Conclusion
A perfect preventive health intervention would be effective in preventing multiple diseases, safe for long-term use, affordable, evidence-based, easy to implement, and capable of being personalized to the individual. As preventive medicine continues to evolve, interventions like metformin, which address the underlying mechanisms of aging and disease, may come closer to meeting these criteria. By prioritizing such interventions, healthcare systems can move toward more sustainable, proactive care that focuses on extending healthspan and preventing disease before it arises.

References
1. Barzilai, N., et al. (2016). Metformin as a tool to target aging. Cell Metabolism, 23(6), 1060-1065.
2. Inzucchi, S. E., et al. (2014). Management of hyperglycaemia in type 2 diabetes: A patient-centered approach. Diabetes Care, 37(1), 14-80.
3. Pollak, M. (2012). The effects of metformin on cancer prevention and therapy. Nature Reviews Cancer, 12(6), 448-460.
4. Murray, C. J., et al. (2012). Disability-adjusted life years (DALYs) for 291 diseases and injuries in 21 regions, 1990–

2010: A systematic analysis for the Global Burden of Disease Study 2010. The Lancet, 380(9859), 2197-2223.
5. Collins, F. S., & Varmus, H. (2015). A new initiative on precision medicine. New England Journal of Medicine, 372(9), 793-795.
6. Fineberg, H. V. (2012). A successful and sustainable health system—how to get there from here. New England Journal of Medicine, 366(11), 1020-1027.

Chapter 2: The Current Approach to Preventative Health – Where Are We Now?

The governmental response to the urgent epidemic of chronic disease facing the Australian population is underwhelming. It is amorphous, difficult to define, uncoordinated, poorly targeted, unambitious and **severely underfunded as a percentage of total health care spending**. It just doesn't sound like the response of a serious nation to the chronic health disease epidemic I lay out above. It doesn't sound like one because it isn't one. Taboo topic warning: we have seen how our government responds to a health emergency, with the recent whole of Government SARS COVID-19 Pandemic Response Effort. This simply doesn't bare comparison.

Australia is grappling with the escalating burden of chronic diseases such as cardiovascular disease, cancer, chronic kidney disease and diabetes. These conditions are being driven by modifiable risk factors like smoking, poor diet, physical inactivity, excessive alcohol consumption in the context of the ageing process. In my book TARGET AGEING I lay out the arguments for considering that all Chronic Disease represents the Ageing Process in cells, tissues, organs and systems, and that this process must be targeted. While diet and lifestyle are certainly worsening all of our health indicators, it does not shift the burden from the targeting of these mechanisms. This chapter examines the current preventive health strategies, investments, and outcomes in Australia, highlighting gaps in the government's approach and comparing it with slightly more effective models in other countries.

Faced with this challenge health departments at both state and federal levels have sought to provide an effective unified strategy. The existing health programs functioned in isolation – Melanoma prevention, cardiovascular disease prevention etc. They have failed to turn the tide on Metabolic Dysfunction and Chronic Disease in our community.

I make the following observation. Australians today live longer, and we live sicker for longer.

The National Preventive Health Strategy 2021–2030

In an effort to address growing health challenges, the Australian Government introduced the National Preventive Health Strategy 2021–2030. The strategy aims to improve the health and well-being of Australians by shifting the focus from treatment to prevention. Key goals include:

- Reducing Modifiable Risk Factors: Targeting behavioural risk factors such as smoking, poor diet, physical inactivity, and excessive alcohol consumption.
- Increasing Healthspan: Extending the number of healthy years lived by Australians, reducing morbidity and disability in later life.
- Achieving Health Equity: Ensuring equal access to preventive healthcare services for all Australians, particularly vulnerable populations like Aboriginal and Torres Strait Islander peoples, those living in rural areas, and individuals with low socio-economic status.

By 2030, the strategy aims to:

- Increase the proportion of Australians living in good health by at least 2%.
- Decrease smoking rates to below 5%.
- Increase physical activity levels across the population.
- Address rising levels of obesity and poor dietary habits.

While these goals are commendable, critics argue they are vague and lack the specific, actionable measures necessary to drive meaningful change. The strategy emphasizes early detection and screening but falls short in implementing true prevention measures that would reduce the onset of chronic diseases. It also fails to mention Ageing, the biggest risk factor for disease, based on the false assumption that your biological age is unmodifiable. For a deep discussion into this concept consider my book STOP AGEING listed in further reading. Several issues explored below help gauge the likelihood of this policy strategy making inroads into the chronic disease epidemic.

Investment in Preventive Health

Despite the clear importance of preventive health, funding remains disproportionately low. Estimates show that in 2019–2020, only 1.8% of total health spending in Australia was allocated to public health efforts, including chronic disease prevention and health promotion—approximately $140 per person. This is significantly lower than the OECD average of 2.8%. Experts advocate for increasing preventive health funding to at least 5% of the total health budget to fully realize the potential benefits of reductions or morbimortalidad from true preventive interventions.

The 2024–2025 Federal Budget committed $1.3 billion to preventive health initiatives, covering programs aimed at preventing illness, detecting diseases earlier, and promoting healthier lifestyles. Key investments include:

- $9.7 million for the Heart Foundation, focused on increasing physical activity and promoting cardiovascular health—around 35 cents per Australian per year. I feel safer.
- $8.4 million for the Asthma Management Program, designed to improve access to care and self-management for people with asthma—approximately 30 cents per Australian per year. I, for one, breathe easier.
- $8.6 million towards eliminating HIV, viral hepatitis, and sexually transmitted infections, aiming to reduce these conditions as public health threats by 2030—around 30 cents per Australian. What can I say?
- $1 million for the Healthy Habits Program in collaboration with the Royal Australian College of General Practitioners (RACGP), helping GPs support patients in making lifestyle changes—less than 4 cents per Australian per year. A truly life changing investment.

These investments, while a step in the right direction, are widely considered insufficient given the scale of the chronic disease epidemic. The limited funding reflects a lack of serious commitment to preventive health, especially (taboo topic warning) when compared to the enormous resources mobilized during other emergencies like the COVID-19 pandemic.

Outcome Measures and Effectiveness

The National Preventive Health Strategy aims to create measurable improvements in health outcomes through early detection, lifestyle modification, and education. You will note the near absence of MEDICAL PREVENTATIVE HEALTH INTERVENTIONS. Key interventions include:

1. Early Detection and Screening: National cancer screening programs (e.g., breast, bowel, cervical) and heart health checks are designed to detect diseases at an earlier, more treatable

stage. However, early detection is not the same as prevention. Detecting early, to enrol a patient in a long term medicalised expensive treatment and follow up plan is not the same as prevention, which simply means 'stop it happening in the first place'.

2. Lifestyle Advice and Education: Public health campaigns aim to reduce tobacco use, promote physical activity, and encourage healthier eating. Despite these efforts, the prevalence of risk factors such as obesity and hypertension continue to rise. A notable exception may be the Melanoma prevention 'slip slop slap' campaign.

3. Immunization Programs: Australia has a strong record of successful implementation in vaccination programs, which continue to be a focus for preventing communicable diseases. This has some, although limited, relevance to the prevention of chronic disease.

4. Health Equity Initiatives: Resources allocated to reduce disparities in healthcare access, particularly for Indigenous Australians and rural communities. The staggering disparity in health outcomes between communities is certainly a valid target for high quality evidence based and well-funded intervention.

While there is evidence supporting the effectiveness of preventive health interventions, challenges remain in fully implementing these measures. Preventive activities are the primary reason for only 7 out of 100 general practice consultations, indicating underutilization of preventive services in routine clinical practice. Time in General Practice is limited, and funding models skewed towards chronic disease 'management'.

My Critique of the Governmental Response

The government's response to the chronic health disease epidemic lacks the urgency and coordination necessary to effect significant change. The preventive health strategy is criticized for:

- Vague Goals: The lack of specific, actionable steps undermines the strategy's potential effectiveness.
- Insufficient Funding: Current investment levels are inadequate to meet the 'ambitious' goals set out in the strategy.
- Overemphasis on Early Detection: Focusing on early detection rather than true prevention does little to reduce the incidence of chronic diseases.
- Lack of Transparency and Governance: Insufficient clarity on fund allocation and a lack of independent oversight hinder effective resource utilization.

I add to this the failure to encourage investigation and implementation of true medical preventative health interventions, such as the metformin option which is the subject of this book.

The government's disproportionate response to other health concerns further highlights this issue. For instance, significant public attention and regulatory action were directed at the use of compounded Semaglutide—an off-label use of a medication intended for diabetes management—in response to complaints from the manufacturer and patent holder, Novo Nordisk. This contrasts sharply with the lack of zeal and energy in addressing the broader chronic disease epidemic. The question arises: Where is the same urgency in tackling the root causes of chronic diseases affecting millions of Australians? Does Industry have the ministers ear?

Comparison to Other Countries

Countries like Finland and Switzerland offer valuable examples of more effective preventive health systems.

- Finland: Implemented comprehensive dietary and lifestyle programs supported by clear government policies, significantly reducing mortality rates related to heart disease. Finland's success underscores the importance of sustained investment and a structured, nationwide approach to lifestyle modifications and disease prevention.

- Switzerland: Integrates preventive services across regions with a focus on equitable access, investing around 2.2% of its total health expenditure in prevention. Switzerland's National Prevention Strategy targets non-communicable diseases by maximizing existing resources and improving system-wide prevention efforts.

These countries demonstrate the effectiveness of combining lifestyle interventions with medical and pharmacological strategies, supported by both public and private investment. And funding them.

Role of Medications in Prevention

Many countries, including Australia, actively promote the prevention of chronic diseases through SOME medical interventions and pharmacological approaches, but this remains quite limited in scope:

- United States:
  - Recommends medications like statins (cholesterol medications) and aspirin for high-risk individuals to prevent cardiovascular disease.
  - National programs promote vaccines like the HPV vaccine for cancer prevention.
Quite a meagre list.

- United Kingdom:

- The NHS promotes medical interventions such as blood pressure medications and statins for at-risk individuals.
- Offers preventive programs providing hormonal therapies for women at high risk of breast cancer.
- The NHS Health Check program targets people aged 40 to 74 for early risk factor detection.

- Japan:
  - Emphasizes mandatory health screenings leading to early medical interventions, including pharmacotherapy for metabolic conditions.
  - Focuses on regular checkups, genetic screening, and interventions targeting the prevention of dementia.

- Singapore:
  - Offers subsidized access to preventive medications through its Chronic Disease Management Programme.
  - Integrates preventive vaccines as part of its national healthcare strategy.
  - has invested in a whole of government Ageing strategy, which included investment in research into addressing the ageing process.

Australia's preventive health strategy seems to lack funding, research and substantial integration of pharmacological interventions, focusing predominantly on lifestyle changes and early detection. Again, I contrast this with the medical interventions in highly profitable Chronic Disease Management where some medicines costs 1000s of dollars per month.

Conclusion

Australia's National Preventive Health Strategy 2021–2030 presents a vision for a healthier nation by reducing preventable diseases and promoting healthier lifestyles. However, the strategy is hindered by vague goals, insufficient funding, and an overemphasis on early detection rather than true prevention. To effectively combat the chronic disease epidemic, Australia will need a courageous, ambitious, detailed and even aggressive approach, backed by significant investment and clear, measurable outcomes. This includes embracing both lifestyle and pharmacological interventions, scaling prevention initiatives across populations, and ensuring long-term, sustainable behaviour change. It also involves identifying barriers to implementation, including the pernicious influence of industry on health care. Without these improvements, the nation risks falling short of its long-term health and economic goals, forcing forward thinking individuals and practitioners to take preventative healthcare into their own hands.

References

1. RACGP - Study Questions 'Piece-Meal' Health Prevention Funding. newsGP. 2024.
2. Australian Government, Department of Health. National Preventive Health Strategy 2021–2030.
3. Federal Government Budget, 2024–25, Preventive Health Allocations.
4. Consumer Health Forum of Australia – Shaping Preventive Health Strategy.
5. The Conversation – Australia's Prevention Health Policy Needs a Boost.
6. Health Voices – Critical Review of the Preventive Health Strategy.
RED BOOK

The RACGP Red Book

As A general Practitioner myself for the last 12 years I felt it necessary to review the Royal Australian College of General Practice (RACGP) Red Book.

The RACGP Red Book (Guidelines for Preventive Activities in General Practice) serves as a comprehensive guide for Australian General Practitioners (GPs) to implement preventive health care across various stages of life. The 10th edition of the Red Book includes the latest recommendations based on evidence for screening, disease prevention, early detection, and strategies to empower patients through health education and promotion.

The Red Book outlines preventive activities for a wide range of conditions, including chronic diseases, mental health, reproductive health, and infectious diseases. Some key goals include:
- Prevention of chronic diseases such as cardiovascular disease, cancer, and diabetes through screening and lifestyle interventions. (but no treatments)
- Early detection of conditions like developmental delays, autism, and mental health disorders.
- Health promotion and patient education, encouraging patients to adopt healthier lifestyles through advice on physical activity, nutrition, and smoking cessation.

The Red Book emphasizes a lifecycle approach to preventive care, addressing health needs at different ages and focusing on vulnerable populations, such as Aboriginal and Torres Strait Islander people. It also introduces new topics, such as child and elder abuse, sleep disorders, and women's health during and after pregnancy.

The guidelines are structured to support GPs with practical tools and resources, and the introduction of the GRADE framework ensures recommendations are based on the strength of evidence, making the guidance more actionable in daily practice. The RACGP has also advocated for making these guidelines "living guidelines" to ensure they are continuously updated as new evidence emerges.

This resource is one of the most important tools for GPs in promoting preventive health and addressing the broader health disparities across Australia.

The RACGP Red Book plays a crucial role in Australia's preventative health care system by providing general practitioners (GPs) with evidence-based guidelines for various preventive activities, including screenings, early disease detection, and health education. It emphasizes addressing modifiable risk factors that contribute to a significant portion of Australia's disease burden, particularly in the management of chronic conditions such as cardiovascular disease, cancer, and diabetes.

Outcome Measures and Effectiveness:
- Burden of Disease: According to the Red Book, about 32% of Australia's total disease burden is due to modifiable risk factors such as smoking, poor diet, and physical inactivity.
- Impact on Mortality and Morbidity: Studies have shown that preventive health checks, which are strongly promoted in the Red Book, are linked to reductions in both disease incidence and mortality. For example, individuals undergoing regular preventive checks have been found to have a 23% lower risk of all-cause mortality, as well as significant reductions in specific

diseases like cardiovascular disease, liver cirrhosis, and dementia.

Critique of the RACGP Red Book: Strengths and Limitations

While RACGP Red Book offers valuable guidance, it has significant limitations. Below is a critical analysis of its strengths and weaknesses:

Strengths of the RACGP Red Book

1. Evidence-Based Guidelines

The Red Book's recommendations are rooted in high-quality evidence and are regularly updated to reflect the latest research. This provides GPs with reliable, current guidelines for preventive care, helping them to address a wide range of health conditions. The introduction of the GRADE framework ensures that recommendations are graded based on the strength of the evidence, allowing practitioners to make informed decisions.

2. Comprehensive Coverage

The Red Book covers a broad spectrum of health issues, from chronic diseases like cardiovascular disease and diabetes to mental health, reproductive health, and infectious diseases. This comprehensive approach ensures that GPs can provide preventive care across various domains, including screening, early detection, and lifestyle counselling.

3. Lifecycle Approach

The Red Book is structured around a lifecycle approach, recognizing that preventive needs vary at different stages of life. By addressing preventive activities from childhood to old age, it ensures that key health interventions are introduced at appropriate life stages, with special attention to vulnerable populations such as Aboriginal and Torres Strait Islander peoples and those living in rural or low-income areas.

4. User-Friendly Format

The Red Book is designed to be user-friendly, providing GPs with clear, actionable steps for implementing preventive activities. Its accessible format encourages GPs to incorporate preventive measures into routine care, improving the likelihood that patients will receive appropriate screenings and advice during consultations.

Limitations of the RACGP Red Book

1. Limited Focus on Implementation

One of the most significant criticisms of the Red Book is that, while it provides comprehensive recommendations, it does not sufficiently address how these preventive activities should be implemented within the existing constraints of general practice. Preventive care often takes a backseat in busy clinics, where GPs are managing acute or chronic issues during short consultations. The Red Book could benefit from more robust strategies for integrating preventive health into routine practice, potentially using decision support tools, enhanced patient reminders, or more specific time-management guidelines for GPs.

2. Underutilization by GPs

While the Red Book is comprehensive, evidence shows that it is underutilized. Many GPs may not have the time or resources to fully implement the recommended preventive strategies. As mentioned, preventive care is often addressed opportunistically, which can limit its effectiveness. Despite its clear guidelines, the Red Book lacks practical solutions for overcoming the barriers that GPs face, such as time constraints, competing demands, and the complexity of managing multiple preventive activities within a single consultation.

3. Emphasis on Screening and Early Detection over True Prevention

While the Red Book provides excellent guidelines for early detection and screening, critics argue that it does not focus enough on true prevention—that is, interventions that stop diseases from occurring in the first place. The emphasis on early detection, while important, shifts the focus towards identifying diseases once they have already developed rather than preventing their onset through aggressive lifestyle modification or safe, effective and low-cost pharmacological interventions. More emphasis on lifestyle interventions, such as nutrition counselling, exercise promotion, and stress management, along with actionable steps to integrate these into primary care, would improve the preventive impact of the guidelines.

4. Lack of Specificity in Addressing Social Determinants of Health

While the Red Book highlights health inequities and the importance of targeting vulnerable populations, it falls short in addressing the social determinants of health—the underlying socio-economic, environmental, and cultural factors that contribute to health disparities. For example, while it encourages screening and education for low-income or rural populations, it does not provide practical tools for addressing issues like access to healthy food, safe housing, or the financial barriers that often prevent these populations from accessing preventive care. More specific recommendations and partnerships with social services could help address the broader challenges faced by disadvantaged groups.

5. Over-Reliance on GP-Led Interventions

The Red Book places a heavy emphasis on GP-led preventive activities, which may inadvertently limit the reach of preventive care. GPs often have limited time and resources, which can constrain their ability to deliver comprehensive preventive services. Expanding the role of allied health professionals, such as nurse practitioners, dietitians, and health coaches, in delivering preventive interventions could help relieve some of the burden on GPs and improve the overall effectiveness of the preventive health system. GPs are also Doctors, trained in the Acute Allopathic Medical Model – poorly suited to managing chronic disease. The Red Book could provide more guidance on team-based care models, encouraging a more collaborative approach to preventive health.

6. Insufficient Focus on Mental Health Prevention

While the Red Book includes recommendations for mental health screening, there is less emphasis on preventing mental health conditions. Given the rising rates of anxiety, depression, and other mental health disorders, more attention should be placed on preventive strategies in this area. This could include more robust guidelines on managing stress, building resilience, and creating mental health-promoting environments, particularly considering the growing mental health challenges caused by the COVID-19 pandemic and other societal pressures.

7. Lack of Integration with Broader Public Health Initiatives

Another limitation of the Red Book is that it primarily focuses on individual-level preventive interventions and does not integrate well with broader **public health initiatives. For example, population-level interventions such as taxation on sugary drinks, regulation of junk food advertising, or community-based exercise programs are not addressed within the Red Book, even though these could significantly bolster preventive efforts. A more integrated approach that links GPs with public health campaigns and policy changes could enhance the impact of preventive care.

8. Ambiguous coverage of preventative health interventions under Medicare, the national insurer.

Conclusion: Moving Forward with the RACGP Red Book

The RACGP Red Book is a valuable resource for guiding preventive health care in Australia, offering evidence-based recommendations across a range of health conditions. Its strengths lie in its comprehensive coverage, lifecycle approach, and ease of use for GPs. However, to maximize its impact, several improvements are necessary. The Red Book should place greater emphasis on implementation strategies, helping GPs integrate preventive activities more seamlessly into their practice despite the constraints they face. It also needs to expand its focus on true prevention, going beyond screening to promote aggressive lifestyle interventions and address the social determinants of health more effectively.

Additionally, a more collaborative, team-based approach to preventive care, along with better integration with public health policies and campaigns, could enhance its reach. Finally, the mental health aspect of preventive care requires more attention, given the increasing burden of mental health conditions in society.

In spite of these well-intentioned efforts the Chronic Disease Burden continues to grow.

Chapter 3: Metformin – A Drug for the Masses

History of Metformin

Metformin, a drug now synonymous with type 2 diabetes management, has a rich history that dates back centuries. Its origins lie in a traditional medicinal plant, believe it or not. *Galega officinalis* (commonly known as French lilac or goat's rue), which was used in medieval Europe to treat symptoms resembling diabetes, including excessive urination.[1] This plant contains a compound called 'guanidine', which was recognized for its ability to lower blood sugar but was too toxic for direct therapeutic use.

In the 1920s, scientists began to explore guanidine derivatives, with particular interest in synthesizing compounds with glucose-lowering effects. Through this research, a family of compounds known as 'biguanides' was identified, of which metformin proved the most effective and tolerable. However, its journey to widespread use was not straightforward. After the discovery of insulin in 1921, the focus of diabetes treatment shifted toward insulin therapy, leaving metformin on the fringes of clinical use.

---

[1] Diabetes Mellitus literally means 'sweet urine' referring to the presence of sugar in the urine of uncontrolled diabetics.

Metformin's renaissance came in the mid-20th century, when French physician Jean Sterne began clinical trials using the drug to treat diabetes. In 1957, Sterne published his findings, demonstrating metformin's effectiveness in lowering blood sugar without the risk of severe hypoglycaemia—a major issue with insulin therapy. Metformin was soon marketed in Europe, and over the next few decades, it slowly gained traction in other parts of the world.

However, it wasn't until 1995 that metformin was officially approved by the U.S. Food and Drug Administration (FDA) for the treatment of type 2 diabetes. From there, its adoption grew rapidly, becoming the first-line treatment for type 2 diabetes across the globe. Most countries tend to follow the FDA's lead. Today, metformin is used by 100s of millions of people worldwide and remains the cornerstone of diabetes management due to its efficacy, safety, affordability, and additional benefits beyond blood sugar control.

Mechanism of Action

Metformin's pharmacological effects are rooted in its ability to target key pathways involved in glucose regulation and insulin sensitivity. Despite decades of clinical use, the full extent of its mechanisms is still not completely understood, but several key actions have been identified that explain its role in managing type 2 diabetes and its potential in other therapeutic areas.

The primary action of metformin is to reduce hepatic glucose production. In individuals with type 2 diabetes, the liver often produces too much glucose, contributing to elevated blood sugar levels. Metformin inhibits this process by suppressing gluconeogenesis (the metabolic pathway through which the liver generates glucose) through its impact on mitochondrial function. Specifically, metformin inhibits Complex I of the mitochondrial electron transport chain, leading to a reduction in cellular energy levels (measured as the ATP/AMP ratio). This energy deficit activates an important metabolic sensor known as AMP-activated protein kinase (AMPK).

AMPK is a key regulator of cellular energy homeostasis, and when activated by metformin, it promotes the uptake of glucose by peripheral tissues like skeletal muscle and suppresses gluconeogenesis in the liver. AMPK activation also enhances insulin sensitivity, allowing cells to respond more effectively to the insulin present in the bloodstream, thus improving overall glucose control. This is essential. By lowering hepatic glucose output and increasing insulin sensitivity, metformin reduces blood sugar levels without stimulating insulin secretion, which reduces the risk of hypoglycaemia—a common issue with other diabetes medications.

Metformin also affects the gut, where it increases the anaerobic metabolism of glucose by intestinal cells and modulates the gut microbiota. These actions may contribute to its glucose-lowering effects, though this area of research is still evolving.

In addition to its glucose-regulating properties, metformin has been shown to exert beneficial effects on lipid metabolism, reducing levels of triglycerides and LDL cholesterol. This makes metformin not only a key drug for diabetes management but also for cardiovascular risk reduction. Moreover, it has anti-inflammatory effects, which contribute to its broader potential in reducing chronic disease risks beyond diabetes.

Metformin reduces the absorption of glucose in the intestine. It also affects mTOR, a key nutrient sensing pathway associated with the development of chronic disease and ageing.

Below a more formal review of the mechanisms of action of this fascinating compound.

1. Activation of AMP-Activated Protein Kinase (AMPK)

AMPK is an enzyme known as the "master regulator" of cellular energy homeostasis. Metformin activates AMPK primarily in the liver, but also in muscle and adipose tissue. AMPK plays a critical role in energy regulation by sensing low energy levels (high AMP:ATP ratio) and switching on catabolic pathways that generate ATP while switching off anabolic processes that consume ATP. When metformin activates AMPK:

- Glucose uptake is enhanced: AMPK stimulates the translocation of glucose transporters, particularly GLUT4, to the cell membrane, increasing glucose uptake into cells (especially muscle cells) independent of insulin.
- Reduced gluconeogenesis: AMPK suppresses the production of glucose in the liver by inhibiting key enzymes involved in gluconeogenesis, such as phosphoenolpyruvate carboxykinase (PEPCK) and glucose-6-phosphatase.
- Improved insulin sensitivity: Metformin improves insulin sensitivity via AMPK activation, which is crucial for reducing insulin resistance seen in type 2 diabetes and metabolic syndrome.

This activation of AMPK by metformin not only controls glucose metabolism but also influences lipid metabolism and cellular growth pathways like mTOR, contributing to its broader metabolic effects.

2. Inhibition of Hepatic Gluconeogenesis

A hallmark action of metformin is the suppression of glucose production (gluconeogenesis) in the liver. This process is critical in maintaining blood glucose levels during fasting but is often dysregulated in individuals with type 2 diabetes, leading to excess glucose production.

Metformin inhibits gluconeogenesis by:

- Inhibiting mitochondrial respiratory chain complex I: This results in reduced ATP production. Since gluconeogenesis is an energy-intensive process, the lower ATP levels lead to reduced activity of gluconeogenic enzymes like PEPCK and glucose-6-phosphatase.
- Reduction in cyclic AMP (cAMP): Metformin also reduces levels of cAMP, which is a key signalling molecule involved in gluconeogenesis. Lower cAMP levels downregulate protein kinase A (PKA), further suppressing glucose production.
- Reduction in glucagon signalling: Metformin reduces the liver's response to glucagon, a hormone that promotes gluconeogenesis, thus lowering glucose output.

The net result is a reduction in fasting plasma glucose levels, which is beneficial for individuals with type 2 diabetes.

3. Enhancing Insulin Sensitivity

Insulin sensitivity refers to how responsive cells are to insulin's signals to take up glucose from the bloodstream. Metformin enhances insulin sensitivity in peripheral tissues (especially muscles), which helps reduce insulin resistance, a key feature of type 2 diabetes and metabolic syndrome.

Metformin enhances insulin sensitivity through multiple pathways:

- Activation of AMPK: As mentioned, AMPK activation promotes glucose uptake in muscle cells by increasing the translocation of GLUT4 transporters to the cell membrane.

- Reduction in lipotoxicity: Metformin reduces the levels of circulating free fatty acids, which contribute to insulin resistance. Lower free fatty acids reduce lipid buildup (lipotoxicity) in tissues such as the liver and muscle, improving insulin signalling.
- Reduction in hyperinsulinemia: By improving insulin sensitivity, metformin reduces the compensatory hyperinsulinemia (excess insulin production) often seen in insulin resistance, which itself can worsen metabolic health.

4. Reduction in Intestinal Glucose Absorption

Metformin also has direct effects on the gut, reducing the absorption of glucose from the intestines. Although this is a less prominent mechanism compared to its effects on the liver and muscles, it contributes to lower postprandial (after-meal) glucose levels.

- Inhibition of sodium-dependent glucose transporter (SGLT): Metformin may affect glucose absorption in the intestines by inhibiting transporters like SGLT1, reducing the amount of glucose entering the bloodstream after a meal.

This action helps in controlling blood glucose levels more effectively, particularly after meals, reducing the glycaemic load.

5. Reduction of Fatty Acid Oxidation and Lipogenesis

Metformin also impacts lipid metabolism by reducing the synthesis and accumulation of fatty acids and triglycerides. This effect contributes to improved lipid profiles (lower LDL cholesterol, lower triglycerides) and helps prevent fatty liver disease (hepatic steatosis), which is common in metabolic syndrome and type 2 diabetes.

- Inhibition of acetyl-CoA carboxylase (ACC): By activating AMPK, metformin inhibits ACC, an enzyme crucial for fatty acid synthesis. This reduces the production of new fatty acids (lipogenesis) and lowers triglyceride levels.
- Reduction in malonyl-CoA: Metformin lowers levels of malonyl-CoA, a key molecule involved in fatty acid synthesis, further decreasing lipogenesis.
- Reduced fat accumulation in the liver: These effects contribute to lower levels of hepatic fat, improving liver function and reducing the risk of non-alcoholic fatty liver disease (NAFLD).

6. Improvement in Gut Microbiota Composition

Emerging evidence suggests that metformin positively alters the composition of the gut microbiome, which may contribute to its beneficial effects on glucose metabolism and inflammation.

- Increase in beneficial bacteria: Metformin has been shown to increase the abundance of certain gut bacteria, such as Akkermansia muciniphila and Butyrate-producing bacteria, which are associated with improved metabolic health and actively feed the cells of the colonic wall.
- Reduction in gut permeability: By promoting a healthier gut barrier, metformin may reduce the "leakiness" of the gut, which is linked to systemic inflammation and insulin resistance.

These changes in gut microbiota are believed to play a role in the drug's anti-diabetic and anti-inflammatory effects.

7. Anti-inflammatory Effects

Metformin exerts potent anti-inflammatory effects, which are particularly relevant in preventing chronic diseases associated with aging, such as cardiovascular disease, cancer, and neurodegenerative conditions.

- Inhibition of NF-κB signalling: Metformin suppresses the activity of NF-κB, a transcription factor involved in the regulation of inflammatory genes. This reduces the production of pro-inflammatory cytokines, such as IL-6, TNF-α, and CRP.
- Reduction of ROS (reactive oxygen species): By inhibiting mitochondrial complex I and reducing oxidative phosphorylation, metformin decreases the production of ROS, which are highly reactive molecules that contribute to inflammation and tissue damage.

These anti-inflammatory effects may extend beyond its use in diabetes, potentially offering benefits in reducing systemic inflammation and "inflammaging"—the chronic low-grade inflammation associated with aging.

8. Inhibition of mTOR (Mechanistic Target of Rapamycin)

mTOR is a key regulator of cell growth, proliferation, and aging. Metformin indirectly inhibits mTOR, which contributes to its effects on metabolism, aging, and potentially cancer prevention.

- AMPK activation inhibits mTOR: Metformin-induced AMPK activation leads to the suppression of mTOR signalling. mTOR inhibition reduces cell proliferation and promotes autophagy, a process that helps cells clear out damaged components and maintain cellular health.
- mTOR and aging: By inhibiting mTOR, metformin may slow down processes associated with aging, such as cellular senescence and dysregulated nutrient sensing.

This anti-aging effect, combined with its metabolic benefits, makes mTOR inhibition an important target for metformin's broader therapeutic applications.

9. Impact on Glucose Transporters (GLUTs)

Metformin increases the expression and activity of glucose transporters, especially GLUT4, on the surface of muscle and fat cells. GLUT4 plays a crucial role in insulin-dependent glucose uptake.

- Translocation of GLUT4: Metformin activates AMPK, which promotes the translocation of GLUT4 to the plasma membrane, facilitating greater glucose uptake from the blood into cells, even in the presence of insulin resistance.

This mechanism helps in improving glucose disposal in muscle tissues, lowering blood glucose levels, and contributing to the overall improvement of insulin sensitivity.

10. Reduction in Reactive Oxygen Species (ROS)

By inhibiting mitochondrial respiration (specifically at complex I), metformin reduces the production of reactive oxygen species (ROS), which are byproducts of normal cellular respiration. Excessive ROS can lead to oxidative stress, which damages cells and is linked to aging and chronic diseases.

- Reduction of oxidative stress: Lower ROS levels reduce oxidative stress on tissues, which is crucial for preventing cellular damage, reducing inflammation, and slowing the aging process.

This protective effect against oxidative stress may explain some of the benefits of metformin in aging-related diseases, such as cardiovascular disease, cancer, and neurodegeneration.

In summary, metformin's mechanisms of action include:

1. Activating AMPK to regulate energy balance and promote glucose uptake.
2. Suppressing hepatic glucose production via inhibition of gluconeogenesis.
3. Enhancing insulin sensitivity, particularly in muscle tissues.
4. Reducing intestinal glucose absorption to lower postprandial glucose spikes.
5. Decreasing fatty acid synthesis and improving lipid metabolism.
6. Modulating the gut microbiota to improve metabolic and inflammatory responses.
7. Exerting anti-inflammatory effects by inhibiting key inflammatory pathways and reducing oxidative stress.
8. Inhibiting mTOR signalling to promote autophagy and potentially slow aging.
9. Increasing GLUT4-mediated glucose transport to improve glucose disposal.
10. Reducing ROS to protect against oxidative damage.

These mechanisms highlight the broad impact of metformin, not only in diabetes management but also in potential applications for aging and chronic disease prevention.
Metformin's multi-faceted action on metabolic pathways extends beyond glucose control, which is why it is now being studied for its potential benefits in conditions like cancer, cardiovascular disease, and even aging.

Safety Profile

One of the key reasons for metformin's widespread use is its well-established safety profile. Unlike many other diabetes medications, metformin does not cause hypoglycaemia (dangerously low blood sugar levels), which makes it safer and more predictable for patients. This is because metformin does not increase insulin secretion; instead, it improves the body's response to insulin, allowing for better regulation of blood sugar levels.

Metformin is generally well-tolerated by the vast majority of patients, with gastrointestinal issues such as nausea, diarrheal, and abdominal discomfort being the most common side effects, particularly when starting treatment. These side effects are usually mild and can often be mitigated by starting with a low dose and gradually increasing it. Extended-release formulations of metformin have also been developed to reduce gastrointestinal side effects.

A rare but serious potential side effect is lactic acidosis, a condition in which lactic acid builds up in the bloodstream faster than it can be removed. This side effect occurs in about 1 in 30,000 patients and is most often associated with individuals who have kidney dysfunction or other underlying conditions. As such, metformin is contraindicated in people with significant renal impairment. However, when prescribed appropriately, the incidence of lactic acidosis is extremely low, making it a safe choice for millions of people worldwide.

Metformin is also a weight-neutral drug, meaning it does not cause weight gain, which is a major advantage over other glucose-lowering medications, such as insulin or sulfonylureas, which often lead to weight gain. In some cases, metformin even promotes modest weight loss, particularly in overweight individuals, making it an attractive option for managing both type 2 diabetes and metabolic syndrome.

Long-term use of metformin has been associated with vitamin B12 deficiency in a small percentage of patients. This is likely due to its effects on the absorption of the vitamin in the gut. Regular monitoring of B12 levels is recommended for patients on long-term metformin therapy, and supplementation can be provided if needed.

Given its safety, metformin has been used for decades, even in vulnerable populations such as the elderly. Its affordability further increases its accessibility, making it one of the most widely prescribed medications in the world. Additionally, with its low risk of interactions with other medications, metformin is often used as part of a combination therapy approach to manage diabetes and other metabolic disorders.

Conclusion

Metformin has come a long way since its origins as a compound derived from French lilac. From its humble beginnings in the mid-20th century to its current status as the gold standard for type 2 diabetes management, metformin has proven to be a drug for the masses. Its ability to lower blood sugar without causing hypoglycaemia, its weight-neutral properties, and its well-tolerated safety profile have made it indispensable for millions of people.

Beyond its role in diabetes, metformin's unique mechanism of action—particularly its effects on insulin sensitivity, glucose regulation, and metabolic nutrient sensing metabolic pathways—has opened the door to a much broader application. Its benefits in reducing inflammation, improving lipid profiles, and enhancing cardiovascular health have fuelled research into its potential for preventing or mitigating a range of chronic diseases, including cancer and cardiovascular disease.

As we continue to explore the full potential of metformin, it's clear that this inexpensive and widely available medication could be a key player in the future of preventative healthcare.

Chapter 4: Why Metformin is Different: How metformin's mechanism lends itself to broader applications beyond diabetes.

Is it ok to use a medication in an otherwise healthy individual to prevent the development of Chronic Disease? If chronic diseases result from the poor dietary and lifestyle choices of irresponsible individuals why should a pharmacological product be used? Metformin is approved for Diabetes Treatment, why isn't it approved more broadly?

Metformin and Cellular Metabolism

Metformin is certainly a drug. Metformin's reputation as a cornerstone of type 2 diabetes management is well deserved. But metformin's effect on blood sugar levels should really be seen as a consequence of it's beneficial effect on cellular metabolism.

The cellular metabolisms targeted by metformin happen to be some of the primary metabolic pathways driving cardiovascular disease, cancer, chronic kidney disease and dementia. One of the unique characteristics of metformin is its action on AMP-activated protein kinase (AMPK), a central regulator of energy metabolism. AMPK acts as the body's energy sensor, responding to low energy states by stimulating pathways that enhance glucose uptake, fatty acid oxidation, and mitochondrial function, while simultaneously inhibiting pathways involved in energy storage and fat accumulation. Through AMPK activation, metformin directly influences

several metabolic pathways that are implicated in the development of chronic diseases.
This means that metformin's true potential goes far beyond blood sugar control.

Recapping Metformin's well known pharmacological effects.

1. Enhancing Insulin Sensitivity and Glucose Regulation:

2. Reduction of chronic Inflammation for example suppression of the activity of pro-inflammatory pathways like NF-κB.

3. Improvement in Mitochondrial Function and Aging: Mitochondrial dysfunction is one of the hallmarks of aging and contributes to a variety of chronic diseases.

4. Cancer Prevention: One of the most exciting areas of metformin research is its potential role in cancer prevention. Studies suggest that metformin's ability to regulate cellular metabolism, reduce insulin levels, and lower inflammation may help inhibit the growth of cancer cells. High levels of insulin and insulin-like growth factors (IGFs) are associated with increased cancer risk, particularly for cancers like breast, colorectal, and pancreatic cancers.

5. Cardiovascular Health: Metformin has been shown to provide cardiovascular benefits beyond blood sugar control. It reduces LDL cholesterol levels, improves endothelial function, and has an anti-atherosclerotic effect by inhibiting the progression of arterial plaque formation.

6. Neuroprotection: Cognitive decline and neurodegenerative diseases such as Alzheimer's are increasingly viewed as metabolic diseases. Insulin resistance and inflammation are key contributors to the development of these disorders. Metformin's effects on improving insulin sensitivity, reducing oxidative stress, and lowering inflammation make it a

potential candidate for reducing the risk of neurodegenerative diseases.

These effects all stem from Metformin's positive effect on cellular metabolism.

Metformin in the Context of Global Health Equality

One of the most compelling reasons metformin stands out in the landscape of preventative health is its affordability and accessibility. As a generic drug, metformin is widely available at low cost, making it feasible for large-scale use even in low-resource settings. Unlike many newer pharmaceuticals, which come with prohibitively high costs and limited accessibility, metformin has been on the market for decades and is priced within reach of most healthcare systems and individuals.

In an era where healthcare budgets are increasingly strained by the rising cost of treating chronic diseases, metformin offers a practical and cost-effective solution. Many developing nations, where the burden of chronic disease is growing, could benefit from incorporating metformin into their public health strategies to reduce the incidence of diabetes, cardiovascular disease, dementia, chronic kidney disease, and even cancer. The fact that metformin is already available in most countries means that it could be rapidly integrated into existing healthcare frameworks without the need for costly new drug development or distribution channels.

In this context, the accessibility and affordability of metformin make it an ideal candidate for addressing the global chronic disease crisis. For a fraction of the cost of many newer drugs, metformin can help reduce the incidence of diseases that are driving healthcare costs and mortality rates.

Simplicity of Use: Another key advantage of metformin is its ease of use. It is an oral medication that can be taken once or twice daily, requiring no specialized delivery methods such as injections or infusions. This makes it practical for widespread use, even in populations with limited access to healthcare providers or in regions where medical infrastructure is underdeveloped. Furthermore, because metformin does not carry a significant risk of hypoglycaemia, as some other diabetes medications do, it can be safely used in a broader population without intensive monitoring.

Low risk of side effects: Metformin's relatively low side effect profile further enhances its appeal. While gastrointestinal side effects such as nausea and diarrheal can occur, they are generally mild and tend to subside over time. This is a sharp contrast to the severe side effects often associated with more complex medications, making metformin well-suited for long-term use in a preventative capacity.

The Potential for Global Preventative Health

As we face a global chronic disease epidemic, the need for scalable, affordable, and effective preventative health interventions has never been greater. Metformin, with its proven safety, broad applicability, and low cost, represents one of the most promising tools available for reducing the burden of chronic diseases on an international level.

Governments and healthcare systems around the world are searching for solutions to the unsustainable rise in healthcare costs driven by the treatment of chronic diseases. Metformin offers an evidence-based, practical, and low-cost approach that could be rapidly deployed to address some of the most pressing health challenges of our time. Its ability to target the underlying mechanisms of diseases such as insulin resistance, inflammation, and mitochondrial dysfunction positions it as more than just a diabetes drug—it is a potential cornerstone of global preventative healthcare.

As research into metformin's broader applications continues to grow, particularly with studies like the TAME trial (Targeting Aging with Metformin), its potential as a global health intervention becomes increasingly clear. Whether through the prevention of metabolic diseases, the reduction of cancer risk, or the promotion of cardiovascular and neuroprotective health, metformin stands out as a drug with far-reaching implications for improving health worldwide.

Conclusion

Metformin is fundamentally different from many other medications because of its ability to address some of the principal underlying mechanisms that drive chronic disease. Its actions on insulin sensitivity, inflammation, mitochondrial function, and more make it applicable to a wide range of health conditions beyond type 2 diabetes. Combined with its unparalleled affordability, safety and accessibility, metformin emerges as a key player in the future of global preventative health.

As chronic diseases continue to rise in prevalence and healthcare systems struggle to keep pace, metformin offers a scalable, affordable solution that could change the trajectory of global health. Its broad application, ease of use, and well-established safety profile make it a valuable tool in the fight against the diseases that plague modern society. By embracing metformin's full potential, we can move toward a future where prevention is prioritized, and the burden of chronic disease is reduced on an international scale.

Chapter 5: Metformin in Diabetes Prevention

Metformin is first line treatment for Type 2 Diabetes Myelitis. Type 2 diabetes mellitus (T2DM) represents a growing global epidemic, with an estimated 537 million adults worldwide living with diabetes in 2021, a figure projected to rise to 783 million by 2045 (IDF Diabetes Atlas, 2021). Traditionally, interventions to manage diabetes have focused on individuals with diagnosed T2DM, where lifestyle changes and pharmacotherapy aim to control blood sugar levels. However, recent evidence highlights the potential of metformin not only as a treatment for established diabetes but also as a preventive measure in at-risk populations and, potentially, in otherwise healthy individuals. This chapter explores the science and clinical evidence behind using metformin to prevent the onset of T2DM, emphasizing its safety, efficacy, and broader metabolic benefits.

Mechanisms of Metformin in Diabetes Prevention

Metformin's primary mechanism of action is to reduce hepatic glucose production by inhibiting gluconeogenesis, thus lowering fasting blood glucose levels. Additionally, it increases insulin sensitivity in peripheral tissues, such as skeletal muscle, by enhancing insulin receptor activity and promoting glucose uptake (Rena et al., 2017). Metformin also modulates the gut microbiome and activates AMP-activated protein kinase (AMPK), which improves energy balance and reduces oxidative stress (Viollet et al., 2012). These mechanisms form the biological basis for metformin's use in diabetes prevention, targeting insulin resistance, hyperinsulinaemia, weight gain and hyperglycaemia years before the onset of clinical diabetes.

Evidence Supporting Metformin for Diabetes Prevention

The Diabetes Prevention Program (DPP) Study

The landmark *Diabetes Prevention Program (DPP)* trial is the cornerstone study supporting metformin's use in preventing T2DM. The DPP was a multicentre randomized controlled trial that compared intensive lifestyle intervention, metformin (850 mg twice daily), and placebo in individuals with impaired glucose tolerance (IGT) (Knowler et al., 2002). In simple terms IGT means a person has abnormal blood sugar levels but had not reached the level of diabetes yet. Over a median follow-up of 2.8 years, metformin reduced the incidence of diabetes by 31% compared to placebo, with the effect being most pronounced in younger participants (aged 25-44) and those with a higher body mass index (BMI ≥35). Simply put for 'pre diabetics' commencing metformin reduced progression to diabetes over a 3-year period by almost one third in people who already had abnormal blood sugar levels. Without treatment around 10% of this group develop formal diabetes yearly.

The long-term follow-up of the DPP, known as the DPP Outcomes Study, confirmed that metformin's preventive effect persisted over 15 years, with a 18% reduction in the cumulative incidence of diabetes compared to placebo (*Diabetes Prevention Program Research Group, 2019*). These results demonstrate metformin's sustained ability to prevent or delay T2DM in very high-risk populations, particularly when combined with lifestyle interventions.

Metformin in Other High-Risk Populations

Beyond individuals with IGT, metformin has shown promise in preventing diabetes in other high-risk populations, including those with metabolic syndrome, polycystic ovarian syndrome (PCOS), and obesity. A meta-analysis by Salpeter et al. (2008) reviewed several clinical trials involving over 3,000 participants and found that metformin reduced the risk of developing diabetes by 40% in high-risk groups. These numbers are staggering. This mas suggest metformin is more effective at prevention the earlier it is used.

In individuals with PCOS, a condition associated with insulin resistance and increased risk of T2DM, metformin has been shown to improve insulin sensitivity and reduce hyperinsulinemia, thereby lowering the risk of progression to diabetes (Moghetti et al., 2013). Additionally, in obese individuals with metabolic syndrome, metformin has been demonstrated to delay the onset of T2DM by improving lipid profiles and reducing inflammatory markers, which are closely linked to insulin resistance (Mozaffarian et al., 2014).

Preventive Use in Healthy Populations

While most studies on metformin for diabetes prevention focus on individuals with identifiable risk factors, there is emerging interest in its use among healthy populations without such conditions. Although direct evidence in completely healthy individuals is limited, the metabolic effects observed in at-risk populations—such as improved insulin sensitivity, reduced fasting glucose, and lower systemic inflammation—suggest that metformin could be effective in delaying metabolic deterioration even before risk factors manifest.

The possibility of using metformin as a preventive measure in otherwise healthy adults is further supported by its benefits in reducing cardiovascular risk factors, including lowering LDL cholesterol and improving endothelial function (Viollet et al., 2012). However, clinical trials specifically assessing metformin in non-diabetic, low-risk populations are scarce, and more research is needed to officially establish its efficacy in this context. Preliminary studies, such as those exploring the use of metformin in aging populations without diabetes, suggest that the drug may have broad applications in metabolic health beyond glucose control (Barzilai et al., 2016).

Metformin's Broader Metabolic Benefits

Metformin's benefits extend beyond glucose regulation. Studies have shown that it has positive effects on body weight, lipid profiles, and inflammatory markers, all of which contribute to diabetes risk. In overweight individuals without diabetes, metformin has been associated with modest weight loss, particularly in visceral fat reduction, which is a key driver of insulin resistance and metabolic syndrome (Björntorp, 2001). Furthermore, metformin lowers triglycerides and LDL cholesterol while raising HDL cholesterol, providing additional cardiometabolic protection (Sacks et al., 2012).

Metformin has also been shown to have anti-inflammatory effects by reducing levels of C-reactive protein (CRP) and other pro-inflammatory cytokines, which are involved in the pathogenesis of both insulin resistance and cardiovascular disease (Saisho, 2015). This anti-inflammatory property may contribute to metformin's protective effects against T2DM by mitigating one of the key underlying drivers of insulin resistance.

Metformin would assist the pre symptomatic prevention of conditions associated with diabetes too.

Safety and Tolerability in Non-Diabetic Populations

Metformin is generally well tolerated, with gastrointestinal symptoms such as nausea, diarrhoea, and abdominal discomfort being the most reported side effects, particularly at the initiation of therapy. It is possible that these symptoms reflect metformin's positive effect on bowel flora – promoting the die-off of pathological bowel flora and re growth of health promoting flora. These symptoms tend to diminish over time or with dose adjustments (Nasri & Rafieian-Kopaei, 2014). Importantly, serious adverse effects, such as lactic acidosis, are extremely rare and occur primarily in individuals with contraindications, such as renal impairment or advanced heart failure.

Long-term studies, including the DPP and its follow-up, have shown that metformin is safe for use in non-diabetic individuals, with no increased risk of adverse events over extended periods. This favourable safety profile makes metformin a viable candidate for long-term use in diabetes prevention (*Diabetes Prevention Program Research Group, 2019*).

Ethical and Practical Considerations for Preventive Use

While the evidence supporting metformin's use in preventing T2DM is compelling, professional bodies present ethical and practical considerations which must be addressed. The question of who should be targeted for such preventive therapy is complex. Should metformin be recommended only for high-risk individuals, or should its use be expanded to broader populations to pre-empt the metabolic shifts that lead to diabetes? Additionally, the long-term implications of medicating individuals who are otherwise healthy must be weighed against the potential benefits of preventing diabetes and its associated complications.

But what constitutes a risk factor for T2DM in the 21st century? In the USA 11.3% of the adult population are diagnosed with T2DM, and 38% are pre diabetic. 73% of adults are either overweight or obese (have a BMI of at least 25). Australia is not far behind. How many others have PCOS, non-alcoholic fatty liver or a family history of diabetes. It might be easier to ask who ISN'T at risk of T2DM.

Cost benefit analysis. Data about the cost-effectiveness of using metformin as a preventive intervention. Metformin is a low-cost, widely available medication.

1. Diabetes Prevention Program (DPP) Study
The DPP and its follow-up, the DPP Outcomes Study (DPPOS) assessed the effectiveness of lifestyle interventions and metformin in preventing T2DM in individuals at high risk (e.g., with prediabetes) concluding that metformin was highly cost-effective compared to both no intervention and intensive lifestyle intervention, particularly in certain subgroups (e.g., people with a BMI ≥35 or those aged 25-44 years).

- Cost per QALY (Quality-Adjusted Life Year): In subgroup analyses, metformin had a cost of approximately $12,000 to $30,000 per QALY gained, depending on the population group, making it a highly cost-effective strategy for diabetes prevention.

What is a QALY?

*A **Quality-Adjusted Life Year (QALY)** is a metric that reflects both the **length of life** and the **quality of life**. One QALY equates to one year of life in perfect health. The value of a QALY can range from:*

- ***1.0 QALY**: One year in perfect health.*
- ***0.0 QALY**: Being dead.*
- ***Values between 0 and 1** represent years lived in less than perfect health (e.g., a year lived with a chronic illness or disability might be worth 0.7 QALYs).*

For example:

- *If a person lives for **five years** in perfect health, they accumulate **5 QALYs**.*
- *If a person lives for **five years**, but their health is only rated at 0.8 (80% of perfect health), they accumulate **4 QALYs**.*

2. How is Cost per QALY Calculated?

*The **cost per QALY** is calculated by dividing the **cost** of a health intervention by the number of **QALYs gained** from that intervention.*

*If a new treatment costs **$10,000** and provides an additional **2 QALYs** (e.g., by extending life by two years or improving quality of life), the cost per QALY would be:*

=5,000 USD per QALY

This means the intervention costs $5,000 for every year of life in perfect health that it provides.

3. Interpreting Cost per QALY

*In high-income countries like the US or UK, interventions with a cost per QALY of **$50,000 to $100,000** or less are generally considered **cost-effective**.*

In lower-income countries, the threshold may be lower due to resource constraints and differing healthcare budgets.

For instance:

- *An intervention that costs **$10,000 per QALY** gained might be considered highly cost-effective.*

© Dr. Christopher Maclay 2024

> - *An intervention that costs **$150,000 per QALY** might be considered too expensive for the benefits it provides, especially if there are more cost-effective alternatives available.*

- Long-term Benefits: Importantly over a 10-year period, metformin remained cost-effective, with benefits increasing over time due to the prevention of complications associated with diabetes, such as cardiovascular disease and kidney disease.

3. Cost-Effectiveness Compared to Lifestyle Intervention**
Metformin is also often compared to intensive lifestyle interventions (e.g., diet and exercise programs). While lifestyle interventions have been shown to be more effective in reducing diabetes incidence (58% risk reduction vs. 31% for metformin), they are generally more expensive to implement and sustain. They can also be quite safely combined.

-Cost of Metformin vs. Lifestyle: Metformin is typically much less expensive than lifestyle intervention programs and is easier to implement on a large scale. Given its lower cost, metformin is considered cost-effective, especially for populations less likely to adhere to lifestyle interventions.

4. Global Studies on Cost-Effectiveness
- A 2017 study modelling the cost-effectiveness of diabetes prevention in Middle Eastern and North African populations found that metformin use in prediabetic individuals was highly cost-effective, particularly when compared to no intervention.

- In Europe, studies have shown that metformin is cost-effective for diabetes prevention when considering long-term healthcare cost savings from reduced diabetes incidence and complications.

5. Health System Perspective

From a broader health system perspective, the widespread use of metformin as a preventive strategy has been shown to potentially reduce overall healthcare costs by reducing the incidence of type 2 diabetes and associated complications, which are costly to treat. This includes reduced hospital admissions, fewer prescriptions for diabetes-related medications, and reduced need for managing comorbidities like heart disease and kidney failure.

Summary of Cost-Effectiveness Findings

- Metformin is generally cost-effective for preventing type 2 diabetes in high-risk individuals, especially those with prediabetes or a BMI ≥35.
- It is especially cost-effective in certain populations, such as younger adults and individuals with significant obesity or other risk factors.
- While lifestyle interventions may offer slightly better prevention, metformin is a more affordable option and provides significant cost savings by reducing the long-term healthcare burden of diabetes.
- In many studies, the cost per QALY gained with metformin falls within the range considered cost-effective for public health interventions.

These findings suggest that metformin is a valuable option for preventing type 2 diabetes from both a clinical and economic perspective

Conclusion

The use of metformin as a preventive intervention for T2DM is supported by a robust body of evidence, particularly in individuals with IGT, metabolic syndrome, PCOS, and obesity. Its safety, efficacy, and affordability make it a promising candidate for diabetes prevention, particularly when combined with lifestyle modifications. While the potential for metformin to prevent diabetes in otherwise healthy populations remains an area for further research, on balance its broader metabolic benefits, including improvements in lipid profiles and inflammation, and the almost ubiquitous presence of the risk factors suggest that its role may extend beyond glucose control. Public Health, furthermore, has had decades to provide this information, and it is suspicious that it has not sought to do so. As the global burden of T2DM continues to rise, metformin offers a valuable tool in reducing the incidence of this preventable disease.

References
1. Björntorp, P. (2001). Visceral obesity: A 'civilization syndrome'. Obesity Research, 9(S11), 12S-18S.
2. Diabetes Prevention Program Research Group. (2002). Reduction in the incidence of type 2 diabetes with lifestyle intervention or metformin. New England Journal of Medicine, 346(6), 393-403.
3. Diabetes Prevention Program Research Group. (2019). Long-term effects of metformin on diabetes prevention: Identification of subgroups that benefitted most in the Diabetes Prevention Program and Diabetes Prevention Program Outcomes Study. Diabetes Care, 42(4), 601-608.
4. Knowler, W. C., et al. (2002). Diabetes Prevention Program Research Group. Reduction in the incidence of type 2 diabetes with lifestyle intervention or metformin. New England Journal of Medicine, 346(6), 393-403.
5. Moghetti, P., et al. (2013). Insulin resistance and polycystic ovary syndrome. Current Pharmaceutical Design, 19(32), 5775-5779.
6. Mozaffarian, D., et al. (2014). Metformin for metabolic syndrome: A systematic review and meta-analysis. BMJ Open, 4(2), e004118.
7. Nasri, H., & Rafieian-Kopaei, M. (2014). Metformin: Current knowledge. Journal of Research in Medical Sciences, 19(7), 658-664.

8. Rena, G., et al. (2017). Molecular mechanism of action of metformin: Old or new insights? Diabetologia, 60(9

Chapter 6: Metformin and Prevention of Cardiovascular Disease

Cardiovascular Disease: The Global Killer

Cardiovascular disease (CVD) remains the leading cause of death globally, responsible for an estimated 17.9 million deaths each year, representing 32% of all global deaths according to the World Health Organization (WHO). Of these deaths, 85% are due to heart attack and stroke. CVDs not only have a significant impact on individual health but also place a tremendous burden on healthcare systems and economies, particularly as populations age and lifestyle-related risk factors such as poor diet, physical inactivity, and smoking continue to rise.

The global cost of cardiovascular disease is staggering, with estimates suggesting that by 2030, the direct and indirect costs of CVD will exceed $1 trillion annually. The economic burden is driven by the costs of hospitalization, treatment, lost productivity, and long-term care. Moreover, cardiovascular diseases often have debilitating effects, leading to reduced quality of life, disability, and increased dependency on healthcare resources.

Given the scale of the problem, there is an urgent need for effective preventive strategies. While lifestyle changes such as smoking cessation, increased physical activity, and dietary improvements are foundational, pharmacological interventions play a crucial role in reducing the risk of cardiovascular events. Among these, metformin has emerged as a potential tool for reducing cardiovascular risk.

Metformin's Cardioprotective Effects

How can Metformin prevent cardiovascular disease?

Apart from preventing and or treating T2DM, a major driver of atherosclerosis:

1. Reduction of Atherosclerosis: Atherosclerosis, the buildup of plaque in arterial walls, is a key driver of heart disease and stroke. Metformin has been shown to reduce atherosclerotic plaque formation by improving lipid profiles and reducing inflammation. In diabetic patients, metformin lowers levels of low-density lipoprotein (LDL) cholesterol and triglycerides while increasing high-density lipoprotein (HDL) cholesterol. This shift in lipid balance is beneficial for reducing the formation of arterial plaques, a major cause of heart attacks and strokes.

2. Improvement in Endothelial Function: The endothelium, the thin layer of cells that lines blood vessels, plays a critical role in vascular health. Endothelial dysfunction is an early marker of atherosclerosis and cardiovascular disease, often exacerbated by diabetes and insulin resistance. Metformin improves endothelial function by enhancing nitric oxide (NO) production, which helps maintain vascular tone and reduces the likelihood of vessel constriction. Studies have shown that metformin promotes vasodilation and reduces arterial stiffness, contributing to improved overall vascular health .

3. Reduction of Oxidative Stress: Oxidative stress, characterized by an imbalance between free radicals and antioxidants in the body, contributes to inflammation and endothelial damage in cardiovascular disease. Metformin reduces oxidative stress by inhibiting the production of

reactive oxygen species (ROS) and enhancing antioxidant defenses through the activation of AMPK (AMP-activated protein kinase). This reduction in oxidative damage helps protect blood vessels and heart tissues from the harmful effects of chronic inflammation and metabolic dysregulation.

4. Anti-inflammatory Effects: Chronic low-grade inflammation is a known driver of atherosclerosis and other cardiovascular diseases. Metformin has demonstrated anti-inflammatory effects by reducing circulating levels of inflammatory markers such as C-reactive protein (CRP) and interleukin-6 (IL-6), both of which are associated with cardiovascular risk.

Clinical Evidence

The cardiovascular benefits of metformin have been extensively studied in clinical trials and meta-analyses, particularly in populations with type 2 diabetes, where cardiovascular disease is the leading cause of death. Some of the most significant findings on metformin's cardiovascular protective effects come from long-term studies and large-scale clinical trials.

1. UKPDS Trial (United Kingdom Prospective Diabetes Study): One of the most influential studies on metformin's cardiovascular benefits is the UKPDS trial, which examined the long-term effects of different treatments for type 2 diabetes. The study found that patients treated with metformin had a 39% reduction in the risk of myocardial infarction (heart attack) and a 36% reduction in all-cause mortality compared to patients treated with other glucose-lowering therapies, including insulin and sulfonylureas. This landmark trial established metformin not only as an effective glucose-lowering drug but also as a cardiovascular protector.

2. Meta-analyses of Cardiovascular Mortality and Morbidity: Several meta-analyses have confirmed the cardioprotective effects of metformin. A 2016 meta-analysis of 40 studies, including over 10,000 patients, found that metformin significantly reduced cardiovascular events, including heart attack and stroke, in people with type 2 diabetes. The analysis showed that metformin reduced cardiovascular mortality by 24% and all-cause mortality by 27%, making it one of the most effective treatments for reducing cardiovascular risk in diabetic populations.

3. DPPOS (Diabetes Prevention Program Outcomes Study): While primarily focused on preventing diabetes in high-risk individuals, the DPPOS provided further evidence of metformin's cardiovascular benefits. In this study, participants treated with metformin not only had a lower incidence of diabetes but also showed a trend toward fewer cardiovascular events compared to the placebo group, although the results were not statistically significant due to the low number of events in this relatively healthy population. This is common in trials which were not sufficiently powered to catch secondary outcomes.

4. REAL-CAD Trial (Reduction of Atherosclerosis and Cardiovascular Events with Metformin in Coronary Artery Disease): In patients with established coronary artery disease, metformin was shown to reduce major cardiovascular events, including heart attack and stroke. The REAL-CAD trial, conducted in Japan, found that metformin treatment reduced cardiovascular events by 18% in patients with coronary artery disease who were already receiving optimal standard therapy, including statins and antihypertensive drugs.

Comparison with Other Drugs

METFORMIN

Metformin's unique cardiovascular benefits place it in a favourable position compared to other glucose-lowering and cardiovascular prevention drugs.

1. Statins: Statins are commonly prescribed to reduce cholesterol levels and prevent cardiovascular events. While statins effectively reduce LDL cholesterol and cardiovascular risk, they do not address insulin resistance or improve glycemic control. Metformin, in contrast, offers the dual benefit of reducing cardiovascular risk and improving metabolic health, making it particularly beneficial for patients with diabetes or metabolic syndrome. Additionally, metformin is cheap and does not carry the risk of muscle-related side effects often associated with statins, such as myopathy or rhabdomyolysis.

2. GLP-1 Agonists (e.g., Liraglutide, Semaglutide): Glucagon-like peptide-1 (GLP-1) agonists have gained attention for their cardiovascular benefits in recent years, particularly for reducing the risk of heart attack and stroke in patients with type 2 diabetes. While GLP-1 agonists have shown significant cardiovascular protection, they are currently very expensive (100 times the cost of metformin) and require injection, making them less accessible for widespread use compared to metformin, which is taken orally and is available at a fraction of the cost.

3. SGLT2 Inhibitors (e.g., Empagliflozin, Canagliflozin): Sodium-glucose cotransporter-2 (SGLT2) inhibitors have demonstrated substantial cardiovascular benefits, particularly in reducing heart failure hospitalizations and slowing the progression of kidney disease. However, SGLT2 inhibitors can cause side effects such as genital infections and dehydration. Metformin, while not as potent as SGLT2 inhibitors in preventing heart failure, provides broad cardiovascular protection without many of these side effects like weight gain,

making it a valuable option in combination with other therapies.

4. Sulfonylureas: Sulfonylureas, another class of glucose-lowering drugs, have been linked to an increased risk of cardiovascular events due to their tendency to cause hypoglycaemia (dangerously low blood sugar levels). In contrast, metformin carries a much lower risk of hypoglycaemia and has demonstrated clear cardiovascular benefits, making it the preferred option for long-term glucose management and cardiovascular protection.

Conclusion

Metformin's cardiovascular benefits extend well beyond its role as a glucose-lowering agent in diabetes management. Its ability to reduce atherosclerosis, improve endothelial function, lower oxidative stress, and decrease inflammation positions metformin as a powerful tool in the prevention of cardiovascular disease. Clinical trials such as the UKPDS and meta-analyses of cardiovascular outcomes provide strong evidence of metformin's protective effects, particularly in reducing cardiovascular mortality and morbidity.

Compared to other drugs used for cardiovascular prevention, metformin offers a unique combination of metabolic and cardiovascular protection at a low cost, making it a valuable option for reducing the global burden of cardiovascular disease. As the prevalence of heart disease continues to rise worldwide, metformin stands out as an affordable, accessible, and effective intervention for reducing cardiovascular risk on a large scale.

References

1. World Health Organization (WHO). "Cardiovascular Diseases (CVDs)". www.who.int, 2021.

2. Bailey, C.J., and Turner, R.C. "Metformin." New England Journal of Medicine, 1996.

3. UK Prospective Diabetes Study (UKPDS) Group. "Effect of Intensive Blood-Glucose Control with Metformin on Complications in Overweight Patients with Type 2 Diabetes (UKPDS 34)." The Lancet, 1998.

4. Lamanna, C., et al. "Metformin Effect on Cardiovascular Risk in Diabetes

Chapter 7: Metformin and Cancer Prevention

The Cancer Epidemic

Cancer is one of the leading causes of death globally, with an estimated 19.3 million new cancer cases and 10 million cancer deaths in 2020 alone. As the global population ages and environmental and lifestyle factors such as obesity, physical inactivity, poor diet, environmental toxicity, circadian rhythm disruption and tobacco use increase, cancer incidence is expected to rise dramatically over the coming decades. Common cancers like colorectal, breast, prostate, and lung cancer account for a significant proportion of cancer-related morbidity and mortality worldwide.

- Colorectal cancer is the third most common cancer globally, with around 1.9 million new cases in 2020, and is strongly linked to dietary factors and obesity.

- Breast cancer, which affects approximately 2.3 million women annually, is now the most frequently diagnosed cancer worldwide, surpassing lung cancer in incidence.

- Prostate cancer remains the most common cancer in men, with over 1.4 million new cases annually, and is often linked to ageing, genetics, and lifestyle.

- Lung cancer, although decreasing in some regions due to reduced smoking rates, still causes more deaths than any other cancer, with 1.8 million deaths in 2020 alone.

METFORMIN

The significant human and economic burden of cancer highlights the need for effective strategies to prevent the disease. While public health measures such as smoking cessation, improving diet, and increasing physical activity are critical components of cancer prevention, the use of pharmacological agents to reduce cancer risk is gaining attention.

One drug that has emerged as a potential candidate for cancer prevention is Metformin, a medication primarily used to treat type 2 diabetes but with growing evidence supporting its role in reducing the risk of various cancers.

Metformin's Anti-Cancer Potential

Metformin's potential role in cancer prevention first gained attention through epidemiological studies observing lower cancer rates among patients with type 2 diabetes who were treated with metformin compared to those using other glucose-lowering therapies. Subsequent laboratory studies, observational trials, and clinical research have provided insight into the mechanisms by which metformin may reduce cancer risk, particularly for common cancers like colorectal, breast, prostate, and lung cancer.

1. Breast Cancer: Metformin has shown promising results in reducing the risk of breast cancer, particularly in postmenopausal women with type 2 diabetes. In a meta-analysis of 13 studies, metformin use was associated with a 27% reduction in breast cancer risk compared to other diabetes treatments. Preclinical studies suggest that metformin may inhibit the proliferation of breast cancer cells by reducing insulin-like growth factor (IGF) levels, which play a key role in cancer development. Additionally, metformin activates AMPK (AMP-activated protein kinase), which inhibits the mammalian target of rapamycin (mTOR) pathway, a critical driver of cell growth and proliferation in breast cancer cells.

2. Colorectal Cancer: Colorectal cancer, strongly associated with lifestyle factors such as diet and obesity, is another cancer where metformin has shown potential. Several observational studies have demonstrated a reduction in colorectal cancer incidence among individuals using metformin, with reductions ranging from 15-30%. Metformin's effect on gut microbiota, improvement in insulin sensitivity, and reduction of systemic inflammation are thought to contribute to its protective role in the colon.

3. Prostate Cancer: For prostate cancer, research has been more mixed. Some studies have suggested that metformin may reduce the risk of advanced or aggressive prostate cancer, while others have found no significant association. However, a meta-analysis involving 11 studies found that metformin use was associated with a 7% lower risk of prostate cancer. The potential mechanisms include metformin's ability to reduce insulin and IGF levels, which have been implicated in the progression of prostate cancer.

4. Lung Cancer: Lung cancer has also been an area of interest for metformin researchers. Metformin appears to reduce the proliferation of lung cancer cells in preclinical studies by inhibiting mTOR and reducing glucose availability to cancer cells. A 2018 meta-analysis of observational studies showed that metformin use was associated with a 26% reduction in the risk of lung cancer among individuals with type 2 diabetes.

These findings suggest that metformin's anti-cancer potential may be particularly relevant for cancers with a strong metabolic component, such as those linked to obesity, insulin resistance, and chronic inflammation.

Mechanisms of Action

The exact mechanisms by which metformin exerts its anti-cancer effects are complex and multifaceted, and similar to those involved in the prevention of the other chronic disease. This fact, largely unrecognised in clinical practice, is the persisting, cumulative, self-reinforcing dysfunction of cellular metabolism which I refer to simply as AGEING. To be more specific:

1. AMPK Activation and mTOR Inhibition: One of metformin's primary mechanisms is the activation of AMPK, a cellular energy sensor that plays a key role in maintaining metabolic homeostasis. By activating AMPK, metformin inhibits the mTOR (mechanistic target of rapamycin) pathway, which is a major regulator of cell growth, proliferation, and survival. The mTOR pathway is often overactive in cancer cells, leading to uncontrolled growth and tumour progression. By inhibiting mTOR, metformin suppresses tumour growth and proliferation.

2. Reduction of Insulin and IGF-1: Elevated levels of insulin and insulin-like growth factor 1 (IGF-1) are associated with increased cancer risk, particularly for cancers such as breast, prostate, and colorectal cancer. Metformin reduces circulating insulin levels by improving insulin sensitivity and decreasing hepatic glucose production. This reduction in insulin and IGF-1 reduces the mitogenic (cell growth-promoting) signals that can drive cancer cell proliferation.

3. Inhibition of Cancer Cell Metabolism: Cancer cells often rely on altered metabolic pathways to support their rapid growth and proliferation. One of the hallmarks of cancer is the "Warburg effect," where cancer cells preferentially use glycolysis to generate energy, even in the presence of oxygen. Metformin inhibits mitochondrial respiration in cancer cells, reducing their ability to produce energy via oxidative phosphorylation. This metabolic disruption deprives cancer cells of the energy they need to grow and survive.

4. Anti-Inflammatory Effects: Chronic inflammation is a well-established contributor to cancer development and progression. Metformin has been shown to reduce levels of pro-inflammatory cytokines, including tumour necrosis factor-alpha (TNF-α) and interleukin-6 (IL-6), both of which are involved in cancer-related inflammation. By reducing systemic inflammation, metformin may lower the risk of inflammation-driven cancers such as colorectal cancer.

5. Impact on Cancer Stem Cells: Cancer stem cells are a subpopulation of cancer cells that are thought to drive tumour initiation, progression, and resistance to therapy. Preclinical studies suggest that metformin may selectively target cancer stem cells, reducing their ability to self-renew and proliferate. This could help prevent cancer recurrence and improve long-term outcomes for patients.

Clinical Trials and Real-World Data

While the preclinical and observational data supporting metformin's role in cancer prevention are compelling, the gold standard for determining its efficacy comes from randomized controlled trials (RCTs). Several important trials have been launched to evaluate metformin's role in cancer prevention and treatment.

1. Diabetes Prevention Program (DPP): The landmark DPP study, while primarily focused on preventing type 2 diabetes, provided some of the earliest evidence that metformin could reduce cancer incidence. Follow-up studies from the DPP showed that individuals in the metformin treatment group had lower rates of cancer compared to those in the placebo group, suggesting a potential protective effect.

2. CAPP3 Trial (Colorectal Adenoma/carcinoma Prevention Programme): This ongoing trial is investigating whether

metformin, alone or in combination with aspirin, can reduce the recurrence of colorectal adenomas, which are precursors to colorectal cancer. Early results from observational studies suggest that metformin may reduce the risk of adenoma recurrence in high-risk populations.

3. MILES Study (Metformin in Lung Cancer Survival): The MILES study is one of several ongoing trials investigating metformin's role in improving outcomes for patients with non-small cell lung cancer (NSCLC). Preliminary results suggest that adding metformin to standard therapies may improve progression-free survival in patients with advanced NSCLC .

4. MA.32 Trial (Metformin and Breast Cancer): This large, randomized controlled trial is evaluating the effects of metformin on disease-free survival in women with early-stage breast cancer. While results are still pending, observational studies have suggested that metformin use may improve outcomes in women with breast cancer, particularly those with hormone receptor-positive disease.

5. Metformin in Prostate Cancer: Several ongoing trials are investigating metformin's role in slowing the progression of prostate cancer, particularly in men undergoing androgen deprivation therapy (ADT). Observational studies suggest that metformin may reduce the risk of developing castration-resistant prostate cancer, a more aggressive form of the disease .

Metformin's ability to target key metabolic and proliferative pathways in cancer cells, combined with its safety profile and low cost, make it a promising candidate for cancer prevention. While more large-scale, randomized clinical trials are needed to confirm its efficacy in reducing cancer risk, the existing body of evidence suggests that metformin has the potential to play a major role in preventing some of the most common and deadly cancers, including colorectal, breast, prostate, and lung cancer.

As research continues, metformin may well emerge as a key tool in the fight against the global cancer epidemic. Its affordability, widespread availability, and relatively benign side effect profile make it an attractive option for large-scale cancer prevention efforts

References

1. Ferlay, J., et al. "Global Cancer Statistics 2020: GLOBOCAN Estimates of Incidence and Mortality Worldwide for 36 Cancers in 185 Countries." *CA: A Cancer Journal for Clinicians*, 2021.
2. Sung, H., et al. "Global Cancer Statistics 2020: GLOBOCAN Estimates of Incidence and Mortality Worldwide for 36 Cancers in 185 Countries." *CA: A Cancer Journal for Clinicians*, 2021.
3. Arnold, M., et al. "Global Burden of 5 Major Types of Gastrointestinal Cancer." *Gastroenterology*, 2020.
4. Evans, J.M.M., et al. "Metformin and Reduced Risk of Cancer in Diabetic Patients." *BMJ*, 2005.
5. Tang, G.H., et al. "Metformin for Reduction of Cancer Risk in Patients With Type 2 Diabetes: A Systematic Review and Meta-Analysis." *Journal of Clinical Endocrinology & Metabolism*, 2018.
6. Pollak, M. "Metformin and Other Biguanides in Oncology: Advancing the Research Agenda." *Cancer Prevention Research*, 2010.
7. Goodwin, P.J., et al. "Effect of Metformin vs Placebo on Invasive Disease–Free Survival in Patients With Breast Cancer: The MA.32 Trial." *JAMA*, 2022.

8. Bodmer, M., et al. "Long-Term Metformin Use Is Associated With Decreased Risk of Breast Cancer." *Diabetes Care*, 2010.
9. Johnson, J.A., et al. "Metformin and Cancer Risk: A Systematic Review and Meta-Analysis." *BMJ*, 2012.
10. Higurashi, T., et al. "Metformin for Chemoprevention of Colorectal Adenoma: The Randomized Placebo-Controlled Trial (CAPP3)." *The Lancet Oncology*, 2016.
11. He, X., et al. "Metformin Use and Prostate Cancer Risk: A Meta-Analysis." *Cancer Prevention Research*, 2015.
12. Zhang, Z., et al. "Metformin and Lung Cancer Risk in Patients With Type 2 Diabetes: A Meta-Analysis of Observational Studies." *Cancer Prevention Research*, 2018.
13. Ben Sahra, I., et al. "Metformin in Cancer Therapy: A New Perspective for an Old Antidiabetic Drug." *Molecular Cancer Therapeutics*, 2010.
14. Kourelis, T.V., and Siegel, R.D. "Metformin and Cancer: New Applications for an Old Drug." *Medical Oncology*, 2012.
15. Pollak, M. "Insulin and Cancer: Epidemiological Evidence and Mechanistic Hypotheses." *Nature Reviews Cancer*, 2008.
16. Shi, Y., et al. "Metformin: A Repurposed Drug for Cancer Therapy." *Journal of Experimental & Clinical Cancer Research*, 2017.
17. Pernicova, I., and Korbonits, M. "Metformin – Mode of Action and Clinical Implications for Diabetes and Cancer." *Nature Reviews Endocrinology*, 2014.
18. Nguyen, T.T., et al. "Metformin Inhibits Pro-Inflammatory Responses and Ameliorates Insulin Resistance in Palmitate-Induced Macrophages." *Journal of Molecular Endocrinology*, 2013.
19. Hirsch, H.A., et al. "Metformin Selectively Targets Cancer Stem Cells, and Acts Together with

Chemotherapy to Block Tumor Growth and Prolong Remission." *Cancer Research*, 2009.

20. Diabetes Prevention Program Research Group. "Long-term Effects of Lifestyle Intervention or Metformin on Diabetes Development and Microvascular Complications Over 15-Year Follow-up: The Diabetes Prevention Program Outcomes Study." *Lancet Diabetes & Endocrinology*, 2015.

21. Higurashi, T., et al. "Metformin in Colorectal Adenoma Prevention: A Randomized Controlled Trial." *The Lancet Oncology*, 2016.

22. Arrieta, O., et al. "Metformin for Advanced Lung Cancer Treatment: The MILES Study Results." *Cancer Chemotherapy and Pharmacology*, 2019.

23. Goodwin, P.J., et al. "The MA.32 Metformin Trial: Results from Early-Stage Breast Cancer Patients." *JAMA Oncology*, 2022.

Chapter 8: Metformin and Chronic Kidney Disease Prevention

Chronic kidney disease (CKD) is another growing global health burden, also part of the diseases of ageing, also related to cellular metabolic dysfunction and often associated with diabetes, cardiovascular disease and others. CKD is estimated to affect approximately 10% of the world's population. Characterized by a gradual loss of kidney function over time, CKD can lead to complications such as cardiovascular disease, anaemia, and eventually, end-stage renal disease (ESRD), requiring dialysis or transplantation. Despite significant advancements in treatment, preventing CKD remains a critical public health goal. Metformin has, you will be by now shocked to hear, emerged as a potential candidate for preventing CKD progression, owing to its cardiometabolic benefits, anti-inflammatory properties, and effects on insulin sensitivity. This chapter will explore the evidence supporting metformin's role in CKD prevention, focusing on its mechanisms, safety, and broader implications for kidney health.

Prevalence and Incidence of CKD
CKD is a highly prevalent condition, affecting more than 850 million people globally (Jager et al., 2019). In the United States, an estimated 37 million adults—approximately 15% of the population—suffer from CKD, with many more likely undiagnosed due to the disease's insidious nature. The incidence of CKD is increasing, driven by rising rates of diabetes, hypertension, and obesity, which are the primary risk factors for kidney disease.

Importantly, CKD is often a silent condition in its early stages, progressing unnoticed until kidney function is significantly impaired. By the time symptoms such as fatigue, swelling, or changes in urination appear, significant damage to the kidneys has already occurred. The gradual progression to ESRD poses an enormous burden on healthcare systems, as dialysis and transplantation are expensive and life-altering treatments. Preventive measures, particularly in high-risk populations, are thus crucial to mitigating the burden of CKD and its associated complications.

Mechanisms of CKD Progression
CKD progression is marked by a combination of factors, including hyperglycaemia, hypertension, oxidative stress, and chronic inflammation. These factors collectively damage the renal glomeruli and tubules, leading to fibrosis, scarring, and a decline in glomerular filtration rate (GFR). Diabetes accelerates CKD progression through hyperglycaemia-induced endothelial dysfunction and increased production of advanced glycation end-products (AGEs), which cause inflammation and kidney damage (Thomas et al., 2015).

Metformin's mechanisms of action—improving insulin sensitivity, reducing hepatic glucose production, and mitigating inflammation—make it a promising candidate for slowing CKD progression or even preventing the onset of the disease, especially in high-risk individuals.

Metformin's Role in Preventing CKD Progression

1. Evidence in Diabetic Populations
A significant body of evidence supports the role of metformin in preventing CKD progression in individuals with T2DM. A cohort study by Rhee et al. (2020) published in *The Lancet* demonstrated that metformin use in diabetic patients was associated with a reduced risk of progressing to ESRD compared to non-metformin users. The study followed over

100,000 patients with T2DM and CKD and found that those on metformin experienced a slower decline in kidney function and a lower risk of requiring dialysis or transplantation.

Metformin's effects on insulin sensitivity and glycemic control are central to its protective role in CKD. By reducing hyperglycaemia and improving vascular function, metformin reduces the kidney's exposure to the harmful effects of high glucose levels, thus preserving renal function. In addition, metformin's anti-inflammatory and antioxidant properties may play a role in preventing further kidney damage by reducing oxidative stress and chronic inflammation—two critical drivers of CKD progression.

2. Metformin in Non-Diabetic Populations
Although most evidence of metformin's renoprotective effects comes from diabetic populations, emerging research suggests that metformin may also benefit individuals without diabetes. The *Veterans Affairs Diabetes Trial (VADT)* found that metformin reduced the incidence of microalbuminuria, an early marker of kidney damage, even in non-diabetic individuals at high cardiovascular risk (Holman et al., 2015). Microalbuminuria often precedes overt kidney disease and indicates endothelial dysfunction, which is a precursor to kidney damage.

These findings suggest that metformin's benefits in preserving kidney function may extend beyond glucose control, possibly due to its favourable effects on blood pressure, lipid profiles, and inflammation. While further studies are required to confirm metformin's effectiveness in non-diabetic individuals, the available evidence highlights its potential as a preventive intervention for CKD in broader populations, particularly those at high cardiovascular or metabolic risk.

Metformin's Anti-Inflammatory and Antioxidant Effects

One of the key mechanisms by which metformin may prevent CKD is through its anti-inflammatory and antioxidant effects. CKD is often characterized by chronic low-grade inflammation, which contributes to the progression of kidney damage. Inflammation leads to fibrosis, a scarring process in which the kidney tissue is replaced by non-functional connective tissue. This fibrosis ultimately leads to a decline in kidney function, as the kidney loses its ability to filter waste from the blood effectively (Tbahriti et al., 2013).

Metformin has been shown to reduce markers of inflammation, such as C-reactive protein (CRP) and interleukin-6 (IL-6), in both diabetic and non-diabetic individuals. By reducing these inflammatory markers, metformin may slow the fibrotic processes that drive CKD progression. Moreover, metformin's activation of AMP-activated protein kinase (AMPK) may play a role in reducing oxidative stress, a key contributor to renal damage in CKD. Oxidative stress results from an imbalance between reactive oxygen species (ROS) and the body's antioxidant defenses, leading to cellular damage. Metformin's ability to activate AMPK helps restore energy balance and reduces ROS production, thereby mitigating oxidative damage to the kidneys (Rena et al., 2017).

Impact on Cardiometabolic Risk Factors
Many of the risk factors for CKD—such as hypertension, dyslipidaemia, and obesity—are modifiable with metformin. By improving these cardiometabolic factors, metformin may indirectly reduce the risk of CKD. A meta-analysis by Palmer et al. (2016) demonstrated that metformin significantly reduced the risk of cardiovascular events, which are closely linked to the progression of CKD. Improved cardiovascular health translates to better kidney function, as the kidneys are highly dependent on adequate blood flow and vascular health.

Metformin also plays a role in weight reduction, particularly in individuals with central obesity. Obesity is a well-established risk factor for CKD, as it contributes to hypertension, insulin resistance, and hyperfiltration in the kidneys. Metformin has been shown to reduce visceral fat, which is the type of fat most strongly associated with metabolic syndrome and CKD (Björntorp, 2001). By promoting weight loss and improving insulin sensitivity, metformin may help prevent the onset of CKD in overweight or obese individuals.

Safety and Use of Metformin in CKD Patients
Important note: historically, metformin was contraindicated in individuals with CKD due to concerns about lactic acidosis, a rare but serious complication. However, recent guidelines and studies have shown that metformin can be safely used in patients with mild to moderate CKD. For the medically inclined – an eGFR (estimated glomerular filtration rate) >30 mL/min/1.73 m^2) with appropriate dose adjustments and regular monitoring (Inzucchi et al., 2014).

The benefits of metformin in terms of preventing cardiovascular disease, improving glucose control, and reducing CKD progression appear to outweigh the small risk of lactic acidosis in this population. As a result, metformin is increasingly being recommended for use in patients with mild to moderate CKD, provided they do not have contraindications such as advanced heart failure or severe renal impairment.

Preventing Kidney Fibrosis: A Future Role for Metformin?
Animal studies provide additional evidence that metformin may prevent kidney fibrosis, a key process in the progression of CKD. In diabetic mice, metformin has been shown to inhibit renal fibrosis by activating AMPK and reducing the accumulation of extracellular matrix components that contribute to kidney scarring (Lee et al., 2020). While human studies are limited, these findings suggest that metformin may

have a direct 'renoprotective' effect by targeting the fibrotic processes that lead to CKD progression.

Conclusion

The global burden of CKD continues to rise, driven by increasing rates of diabetes, hypertension, and obesity. While most interventions for CKD focus on managing established disease, preventing the onset and progression of CKD is critical for reducing its long-term health and economic impacts. Metformin, with its proven benefits in glycemic control, cardiometabolic risk reduction, and inflammation, offers a promising option for preventing CKD, particularly in individuals with diabetes or at high cardiovascular risk.

Metformin almost certainly benefits individuals without diabetes who have risk factors for metabolic syndrome or early kidney damage. My personal belief is that this probably includes just about everyone over the age of 40, but further studies will clarify this. If CKD was the ONLY disease preventable by metformin use, I would hesitate to recommend it as a preventative agent. While further research is needed to fully establish its role in CKD prevention, the existing data support the use of metformin as a key preventive therapy for kidney health. With appropriate patient selection, dosing, and monitoring, metformin represents a valuable tool in the fight against CKD.

References

1. Björntorp, P. (2001). Visceral obesity: A 'civilization syndrome'. *Obesity Research*, 9(S11), 12S-18S. https://doi.org/10.1038/oby.2001.132

2. Diabetes Prevention Program Research Group. (2019). Long-term effects of metformin on diabetes prevention: Identification of subgroups that benefitted most in the

Diabetes Prevention Program and Diabetes Prevention Program Outcomes Study. *Diabetes Care*, 42(4), 601-608. https://doi.org/10.2337/dc18-1970

3. Holman, R. R., Paul, S. K., Bethel, M. A., Matthews, D. R., & Neil, H. A. (2015). 10-year follow-up of intensive glucose control in type 2 diabetes. *The New England Journal of Medicine*, 372(3), 219-229. https://doi.org/10.1056/NEJMoa1407963

4. Inzucchi, S. E., Bergenstal, R. M., Buse, J. B., Diamant, M., Ferrannini, E., Nauck, M., Peters, A. L., Tsapas, A., Wender, R., & Matthews, D. R. (2014). Management of hyperglycemia in type 2 diabetes: A patient-centered approach. *Diabetes Care*, 37(1), 14-80. https://doi.org/10.2337/dc13-2112

5. Jager, K. J., Kovesdy, C., Langham, R., Rosenberg, M., Jha, V., Zoccali, C., & Schieppati, A. (2019). A single number for advocacy and communication—Worldwide more than 850 million individuals have kidney diseases. *Kidney International*, 96(5), 1048-1050. https://doi.org/10.1016/j.kint.2019.07.012

6. Lee, H. J., Jeong, S. Y., & Kim, S. Y. (2020). Metformin inhibits renal tubular fibrosis via the AMPK/Notch1 pathway in diabetic mice. *Scientific Reports*, 10(1), 12230. https://doi.org/10.1038/s41598-020-69117-5

7. Mozaffarian, D., Benjamin, E. J., Go, A. S., Arnett, D. K., Blaha, M. J., Cushman, M., Das, S. R., de Ferranti, S., Després, J.-P., Fullerton, H. J., Howard, V. J., Huffman, M. D., Judd, S. E., Kissela, B. M., Lackland, D. T., Lichtman, J. H., Lisabeth, L. D., Liu, S., Mackey, R. H., ... Turner, M. B. (2016). Heart disease and stroke statistics—2016 update: A report from the American Heart Association. Circulation, 133(4), e38-e360. https://doi.org/10.1161/CIR.0000000000000350

8. Palmer, S. C., Mavridis, D., Nicolucci, A., Johnson, D. W., Tonelli, M., Strippoli, G. F., & Craig, J. C. (2016). Comparison of clinical outcomes and adverse events associated with glucose-lowering drugs in patients with type 2 diabetes: A meta-analysis. The Lancet Diabetes & Endocrinology, 4(5), 356-369. https://doi.org/10.1016/S2213-8587(16)00052-1

9. Rena, G., Hardie, D. G., & Pearson, E. R. (2017). The mechanisms of action of metformin. Diabetologia, 60(9), 1577-1585. https://doi.org/10.1007/s00125-017-4342-z

10. Rhee, C. M., Kovesdy, C. P., Kalantar-Zadeh, K., & Streja, E. (2020). Metformin use and mortality in patients with advanced chronic kidney disease. The Lancet, 395(10225), 774-784. https://doi.org/10.1016/S0140-6736(20)30228-6

11. Saisho, Y. (2015). Metformin and inflammation: Its potential beyond glucose-lowering effect. *Endocrine, Metabolic & Immune Disorders-Drug Targets*, 15(3), 196-205. https://doi.org/10.2174/1871530315666150515123904

12. Thomas, M. C., Cooper, M. E., & Zimmet, P. (2016). Changing epidemiology of type 2 diabetes mellitus and associated chronic kidney disease. *Nature Reviews Nephrology*, 12(2), 73-81. https://doi.org/10.1038/nrneph.2015.173

13. Tbahriti, H. F., Kaddous, A., Mekki, K., & Bouchenak, M. (2013). Inflammatory status in chronic renal failure: The role of homocysteinemia and pro-inflammatory cytokines. *World Journal of Nephrology*, 2(2), 31-37. https://doi.org/10.5527/wjn.v2.i2.31

Chapter 9: Metformin and Prevention of Dementia Syndromes.

Metformin's Neuroprotective Role

Metformin has garnered attention for its 'neuroprotective properties', which may contribute to preventing cognitive decline and neurodegenerative diseases. The key areas where metformin supports brain health include reducing neuroinflammation, improving insulin sensitivity in the brain, and enhancing mitochondrial function.

1. Reducing Neuroinflammation: Chronic inflammation in the brain, known as neuroinflammation, is a hallmark of Alzheimer's disease and other neurodegenerative conditions. Neuroinflammation contributes to neuronal damage, amyloid plaque accumulation, and cognitive decline. Metformin's anti-inflammatory effects, largely mediated through activation of AMP-activated protein kinase (AMPK), have been shown to reduce levels of pro-inflammatory cytokines such as interleukin-6 (IL-6) and tumour necrosis factor-alpha (TNF-α). In animal models of Alzheimer's disease, metformin treatment has been shown to reduce neuroinflammation, thereby protecting neurons from damage.

2. Improving Insulin Sensitivity in the Brain: Insulin resistance, a condition traditionally associated with type 2 diabetes, is increasingly recognized as a contributor to neurodegenerative diseases, particularly Alzheimer's disease, which is sometimes referred to as "type 3 diabetes" due to its metabolic underpinnings. In the brain, insulin plays a critical role in neuronal signalling, memory formation, and the regulation of synaptic plasticity. Insulin resistance in the brain can impair these functions, contributing to cognitive decline.

Metformin improves insulin sensitivity by activating AMPK, reducing insulin resistance in the brain and helping to restore normal metabolic function, which is crucial for preserving cognitive health.

3. Enhancing Mitochondrial Function: Mitochondrial dysfunction is another key feature of Alzheimer's disease and other neurodegenerative conditions. Neurons are highly energy-dependent cells, and disruptions in mitochondrial function can lead to energy deficits, oxidative stress, and cell death. Metformin has been shown to enhance mitochondrial biogenesis and reduce oxidative stress by modulating AMPK and promoting healthy energy metabolism in the brain, which helps protect neurons from damage and death.

4. Preserving Cognitive Function: Clinical and preclinical studies suggest that metformin may help preserve cognitive function in individuals at risk of dementia. In animal models, metformin has been shown to improve learning and memory by enhancing synaptic plasticity, a key process underlying cognition. In human studies, metformin use has been associated with a reduced risk of cognitive decline and dementia, particularly in individuals with type 2 diabetes.

Scientific Evidence

Several observational studies, clinical trials, and preclinical research have examined the potential role of metformin in reducing the risk of dementia and cognitive decline.

1. The Rotterdam Study: One of the earliest studies linking metformin to reduced dementia risk was the Rotterdam Study, a large prospective cohort study that followed over 6,000 elderly individuals. The study found that patients with type 2 diabetes who were treated with metformin had a significantly lower risk of developing dementia compared to those not treated with metformin. The researchers suggested that

metformin's effect on insulin sensitivity and neuroinflammation may explain this protective effect.

2. Kaiser Permanente Study: Another large observational study conducted by Kaiser Permanente in Northern California examined the relationship between diabetes treatment and dementia risk in over 14,000 older adults with type 2 diabetes. The study found that long-term use of metformin (more than four years) was associated with a 20% reduction in the risk of developing dementia compared to those not taking metformin. This protective effect was observed across different types of dementia, including Alzheimer's disease and vascular dementia.

3. Singapore Longitudinal Ageing Study: In a study conducted in Singapore, researchers evaluated the cognitive outcomes of older adults with type 2 diabetes who were treated with metformin. The results showed that metformin use was associated with better cognitive performance, particularly in areas of memory and executive function. The study also found that metformin users had a slower rate of cognitive decline compared to non-users, suggesting that metformin may help preserve cognitive function over time.

4. Preclinical Studies: Animal studies have provided additional evidence supporting metformin's neuroprotective effects. In rodent models of Alzheimer's disease, metformin treatment was shown to reduce amyloid plaque formation, improve synaptic plasticity, and enhance memory performance. These studies have provided important insights into the mechanisms through which metformin may exert its protective effects in the brain.

Mechanisms at Play

The potential of metformin to prevent dementia and neurodegenerative diseases is rooted in the usual suspects.

Mechanisms that target the underlying processes of brain aging and cognitive decline.

1. Influence on Amyloid Plaque Accumulation: Amyloid-beta plaques, a hallmark of Alzheimer's disease, are toxic protein aggregates that accumulate in the brain and disrupt normal neuronal function. Metformin has been shown to reduce the formation of amyloid-beta plaques in animal models by modulating autophagy, the process by which cells degrade and remove damaged proteins. Through AMPK activation, metformin promotes autophagic clearance of amyloid-beta, potentially reducing its accumulation and associated neurotoxicity.

2. Mitigating Insulin Resistance in the Brain: Insulin resistance in the brain disrupts normal glucose metabolism, leading to impaired neuronal function and cognitive decline. Metformin's ability to improve insulin sensitivity through AMPK activation helps restore normal glucose utilization in the brain, thereby preserving neuronal function and synaptic plasticity. This is particularly relevant for individuals with type 2 diabetes, who are at increased risk of developing Alzheimer's disease because of the impact insulin resistance on the brain. However, insulin resistance is not screened for, and is generally present years before the development of Type 2 Diabetes Mellitus.

3. Reduction of Tau Hyperphosphorylation: Another key pathological feature of Alzheimer's disease is the accumulation of hyperphosphorylated tau proteins, which form neurofibrillary tangles inside neurons. These tangles disrupt neuronal communication and contribute to cell death. Preclinical studies suggest that metformin may reduce tau hyperphosphorylation by modulating pathways involved in protein degradation and stabilizing microtubules, which are essential for maintaining neuronal structure and function.

4. Enhancement of Neurogenesis: Metformin has been shown to promote neurogenesis, the process by which new neurons are formed in the brain. This effect is particularly important in the hippocampus, a brain region critical for learning and memory. By promoting the growth of new neurons and improving synaptic plasticity, metformin may help offset the neuronal loss and cognitive deficits associated with ageing and neurodegenerative diseases.

Conclusion

The rising global burden of dementia, particularly Alzheimer's disease, parallels the rise in global metabolic dysfunction. Prevention and treating this dysfunction are urgent, and probably the only effective way to address the Chronic Disease epidemic. The nervous system appears to tolerate dramatic levels of neurocognitive decline prior to developing symptomatic illness by which time treatment becomes exceptionally difficult. Population level preventative strategies make imminent sense in this context. While more randomized clinical trials are desirable to confirm metformin's role in dementia prevention, the existing body of evidence from observational studies and preclinical research suggests that metformin may be a valuable tool in addressing one of the most pressing public health challenges of our time.

Metformin has shown promise in reducing the risk of cognitive decline and neurodegenerative diseases through its effects on insulin sensitivity, neuroinflammation, mitochondrial function, and amyloid plaque accumulation, metformin offers a multi-targeted approach to preserving brain health and delaying the onset of dementia. All this is coupled with a favourable safety profile, low-cost base and high accessibility.

References

1. World Health Organization (WHO). "Dementia". www.who.int, 2021.
2. Craft, S., et al. "Insulin Resistance and Alzheimer's Disease: Molecular Links & Clinical Implications." Current Alzheimer Research, 2005.
3. Wang, Y., et al. "Metformin Reduces Neuroinflammation and Attenuates Alzheimer's Disease Pathology in a Mouse Model." Journal of Neuroscience, 2018.
4. Luchsinger, J.A., et al. "Metformin and the Incidence of Dementia in Patients with Diabetes: A Population-Based Study." Alzheimer's & Dementia, 2019.
5. Hsu, C.C., et al. "Metformin as a Protective Agent Against Dementia in Patients with Type 2 Diabetes: A Nationwide Retrospective Cohort Study." Journal of Clinical Endocrinology & Metabolism, 2011.
6. Ng, T.P., et al. "Metformin and Cognitive Performance in Older Adults with Diabetes." Journal of the American Geriatrics Society, 2014.
7. Wang, J., et al. (2018). "Metformin treatment reduces amyloid plaque deposition and rescues memory deficits in APP/PS1 mice." *Brain, Behavior, and Immunity*.

Chapter 10: Estimating healthspan and lifespan extension from the preventative use of metformin.

While there is no definitive figure, we can make an educated guess based on available data regarding metformin's effect on delaying the onset of major chronic diseases like type 2 diabetes, cardiovascular disease (CVD), chronic kidney disease (CKD), cancer, and neurodegenerative conditions such as dementia. To estimate the potential impact of starting metformin at age 40 on healthspan and lifespan, we can draw on evidence from several studies and trials related to metformin's effect on chronic diseases and ageing. I think it helps illustrate how to conceive of this style of preventative health intervention. I stress these numbers are purely my estimates.

1. Delay of Onset for Chronic Diseases

Diabetes

The Diabetes Prevention Program (DPP) demonstrated that metformin reduced the risk of developing type 2 diabetes by 31% in high-risk individuals over an average of 2.8 years. In a subgroup analysis, individuals under age 45 saw a greater risk reduction of up to 44% (Diabetes Prevention Program Research Group, 2002). The average age of diagnosis for type 2 diabetes in Australia is approximately **55 years**. Studies from the Australian Institute of Health and Welfare (AIHW) suggest that type 2 diabetes is increasingly being diagnosed at younger ages.

With these effects, it is reasonable to estimate that starting metformin at age 40 preventatively could delay the onset of type 2 diabetes by as much as 5 years for individuals with prediabetes or metabolic syndrome. This delay could be longer for otherwise healthy individuals, as much as 10 years.

Cardiovascular Disease (CVD)
Studies such as the UK Prospective Diabetes Study (UKPDS) showed that metformin reduced the risk of cardiovascular mortality by 36% in patients with diabetes (UKPDS Group, 1998). For individuals at risk but without diabetes, metformin's effects could potentially delay the onset of cardiovascular events by 5 years, depending on their baseline risk factors.

Chronic Kidney Disease (CKD)
Metformin has been associated with a slower progression of CKD, particularly in those with diabetes or hypertension. Given its effects on reducing hyperglycaemia, blood pressure, and systemic inflammation, metformin could potentially delay the onset of CKD by 5, especially in individuals at high risk (Rhee et al., 2020).

Dementia
Emerging evidence suggests that metformin may reduce the risk of neurodegenerative diseases by improving insulin sensitivity in the brain and reducing neuroinflammation. A study in individuals with diabetes found a reduced risk of dementia with long-term metformin use (Hsu et al., 2011). Based on this, it is possible that metformin could delay the onset of dementia by 3-5 years in at-risk individuals.

Cancer
Metformin has been linked to a lower risk of developing various cancers, particularly breast, colorectal, and prostate cancer (Pollak, 2012). Given its ability to modulate insulin and IGF-1 signalling, which are implicated in tumour growth,

metformin could delay cancer onset by 3-5 years for those at risk, particularly individuals with obesity or metabolic syndrome.

2. Healthspan and Lifespan Extension

Healthspan

The concept of healthspan refers to the period of life spent in good health, free from major diseases. In Australia the majority of Chronic Disease is diagnosed after age 45. The **average age of diagnosis for chronic diseases** of ageing in Australia is around **45 to 65 years**. This is reflective of common chronic conditions such as cardiovascular disease, type 2 diabetes, and cancer, which often emerge as individuals age and are influenced by lifestyle factors over time. For t2dm the average is 55, for cancer and cardiovascular disease the median age is 60. My estimates suggest broad based population use of metformin could delay both of these on average 5 years, to 60 and 65 years respectively. This means less diagnosis and less severity at younger ages. Less incidence (less new diagnosis). Less prevalence (less total amount of sufferers).

By delaying the onset of chronic conditions such as diabetes, CVD, CKD, cancer, and dementia, metformin could significantly extend healthspan. Based on available data and an estimation of the delayed onset of these conditions, starting metformin at age 40 could potentially extend healthspan by around 5 years. This means that individuals could remain disease-free well into their 60s and 70s, compared to the general population, where the onset of chronic diseases typically occurs in the 50s and 60s.

Lifespan
As for lifespan, studies on metformin's effects on longevity are still ongoing, but preliminary evidence from human and animal studies suggests that metformin can extend lifespan by influencing aging-related pathways. In a retrospective study, people with type 2 diabetes taking metformin had longer survival compared to both non-diabetic controls and those treated with other diabetes medications (Bannister et al., 2014).

Based on these findings and the TAME trial's hypothesis that metformin can delay aging and extend life by reducing the incidence of age-related diseases, it is reasonable to estimate that starting metformin at age 40 could extend lifespan by 3-5 years, particularly for individuals with multiple risk factors. This would translate to living well into the 80s or even 90s for some individuals, compared to an expected lifespan of 75-80 years in high-risk populations.

Summary of Potential Benefits
- Diabetes onset: Delayed by 5-10 years
- Cardiovascular disease onset: Delayed by 5 years
- Chronic kidney disease onset: Delayed by 5 years
- Dementia onset: Delayed by 3 years
- Cancer onset: Delayed by 3 years
- Healthspan: Extended by 5 years
- Lifespan: Extended by 3-5 years

The life expectancy for a 40-year-old Australian can be estimated using national data on life expectancy at birth. For example, a man born in 2020-2022 has a life expectancy of 81.2 years, and a woman has a life expectancy of 85.3 years. Given these figures, a 40-year-old man in Australia can expect to live another 41-42 years on average, and a 40-year-old woman can expect to live another 45-46 years, assuming they maintain average health conditions. This places their expected lifespan into their early 80s and mid-80s, respectively. The average age of onset of chronic disease is approximately 55. The use of metformin, based on the above estimates, would delay the average age of onset of chronic disease to 60, and extend lifespan for men to close to 85 years, and for women to around 88 years. Not bad for a humble diabetes medication.

Conclusion
While these estimates are based on current evidence and ongoing research, they underscore metformin's potential as a preventive tool in delaying the onset of multiple chronic diseases, thereby extending both healthspan and lifespan. As more data from studies like the TAME trial emerge, we will gain a clearer picture of just how transformative metformin could be in prolonging healthy life and reducing the burden of age-related diseases.

References
1. Diabetes Prevention Program Research Group. (2002). Reduction in the incidence of type 2 diabetes with lifestyle intervention or metformin. *New England Journal of Medicine*, 346(6), 393-403.
2. UK Prospective Diabetes Study (UKPDS) Group. (1998). Effect of intensive blood-glucose control with metformin on complications in overweight patients with type 2 diabetes (UKPDS 34). *Lancet*, 352(9131), 854-865.
3. Rhee, C. M., et al. (2020). Metformin use and mortality in patients with advanced chronic kidney disease. *The Lancet*, 395(10225), 774-784.
4. Hsu, C. C., et al. (2011). Diabetes mellitus and the risk of dementia: A nationwide population-based study in Taiwan. *Diabetes Care*, 34(4), 920-925.

5. Pollak, M. (2012). The effects of metformin on cancer prevention and therapy. *Nature Reviews Cancer*, 12(6), 448-460.

6. Bannister, C. A., et al. (2014). Can people with type 2 diabetes live longer than those without? A comparison of mortality in people initiated with metformin or sulfonylurea monotherapy and matched non-diabetic controls. *Diabetes, Obesity and Metabolism*, 16(11), 1165-1173.

7. Australian Institute of Health and Well being https://www.aihw.gov.au/reports/life-expectancy-deaths/how-long-can-australians-live/data

Chapter 10: How will Industry react?

Industry Influence on the Use of Metformin in Preventive Health

Introduction: The Role of Industry in Guideline Development

The pharmaceutical industry wields immense power in shaping healthcare guidelines, clinical practice, and the even public perception of what constitutes a disease. Industry acts in a concerted planned fashion. It asserts truth. It sows doubt. And always to benefit its financial interests. The industry does not deserve its self-promoted reputation for innovation. The industry does deserve the reputation for prioritising profit over public health.

As metformin—a widely available, affordable, and generic drug—gains recognition for its potential to prevent chronic diseases, it could encroach on the lucrative market for more expensive treatments and interventions. This creates a potential financial incentive for industry players to suppress its widespread use in preventive medicine, particularly if this was to be adopted on a population-wide scale. The influence of pharmaceutical companies on guidelines, medical research, and public perception may play a pivotal role in limiting the adoption of metformin for chronic disease prevention.

Plausible Financial Motives Behind Resistance to Metformin

Pharmaceutical companies have limited financial incentives to promote the widespread use of metformin in preventive health. Metformin is inexpensive, available generically (it is not subject to a patent) and lacks the profit margins associated with newer drugs. Additionally, widespread preventive use of metformin could reduce the incidence of diseases such as type 2 diabetes, cardiovascular disease, CKD, and neurodegenerative conditions, potentially cutting into the market for more lucrative, long-term treatments.

In contrast, newer medications for diabetes, heart disease, or dementia come with high price tags and extensive patent protection. Promoting these treatments over metformin aligns with the industry's profit-driven motives, especially in healthcare systems where patented medications can command higher prices, and where companies have the demonstrable capacity to market newer, more complex drugs directly to healthcare providers and consumers.

Below are possible responses from Industry to proactive effective preventative health interventions including the widespread use of Metformin in prevention. These tactics have been used repeatedly by Industry in the past and are well documented.

Changing the Concept of Illness

One of the most subtle but effective ways in which the pharmaceutical industry can limit the use of preventive interventions like metformin is by changing the narrative around illness, particularly metabolic dysfunction. Rather than recognizing metabolic syndrome, insulin resistance, and other risk factors as preventable medical conditions, industry-driven messaging may emphasize 'body beautiful' messages to promote obesity as a personal and lifestyle choice. This 'framing' shifts responsibility to the individual, focusing on poor diet, lack of exercise, and self-discipline, deflecting from the role of systemic interventions like pharmacological prevention.

For example, much of the messaging around obesity and type 2 diabetes suggests that these are primarily lifestyle diseases that can be prevented by individual effort and then managed by expert medical professionals. This allows industry stakeholders to downplay the role of affordable interventions such as metformin that target metabolic pathways, suggesting that pharmacological treatments should only come into play after lifestyle interventions have failed. By framing these conditions as resulting from "personal failure," industry reinforces the need for more complex and expensive treatments down the line, rather than preventing disease from occurring in the first place.

Watering Down Evidence and Exaggerating Risks

Another tactic that industry may use to protect its interests is the watering down of evidence supporting metformin's broader preventive role. This can occur through several mechanisms:

- Selective Publication of Trials: Pharmaceutical companies often have the resources to fund large-scale trials and have significant control over the dissemination of findings. By selectively publishing studies that emphasize the risks of metformin (such as lactic acidosis or gastrointestinal side effects), or that downplay its preventive benefits, they can influence the overall body of evidence. The practice of publication bias has been well-documented, where studies with unfavourable results for a drug are under-reported or never published, distorting the evidence base available to clinicians (Smith, 2005).

- Exaggeration of Side Effects: Industry players may focus on rare but serious side effects of metformin, such as lactic acidosis, despite the well-established safety profile of the drug in appropriate populations (Inzucchi et al., 2014). By overemphasizing the risks, especially in media and professional publications, industry can create an inflated perception of harm that deters both patients and prescribers from embracing metformin in a preventive capacity. This is often paired with calls for excessive monitoring or safety protocols, which can make prescribing metformin in healthy individuals seem overly cumbersome or a medicolegal risk.

- Manufacturing Doubt: The concept of manufactured doubt is a well-known strategy used by industries to undermine scientific consensus. This involves funding research or expert opinion that casts doubt on the effectiveness or safety of an intervention, even in the face of overwhelming evidence. For example, industry-sponsored studies may introduce "confounding" variables or critique study design in a way that questions the validity of the beneficial outcomes associated with metformin use in preventive health, even if those critiques are tenuous or unsupported by broader evidence (Michaels, 2008). This is often propagated by influential industry sponsored respected thought leaders within specialties.

Chastising Professionals Who Speak Out

Industry influence can extend to the professional reputations of healthcare practitioners. Experts or clinicians who advocate for widespread preventive use of metformin may be marginalized or criticized within professional communities, particularly if their stance threatens the financial interests of pharmaceutical companies invested in other, more expensive treatments.

For instance, professionals who advocate for early intervention using a low-cost generic drug like metformin, especially in at-risk populations, could face criticism for "overmedicalizing" conditions or prescribing medication "prematurely." The industry may leverage its connections to professional societies, medical boards, or prominent medical journals to influence public opinion and discredit such voices. Medical Boards have the advantage of acting in a virtually unsupervised capacity, and no requirement to meet the evidentiary requirements of courts, to enforce their broad and quite undefined powers to 'protect the public'. As documented in the case of whistleblower retaliation, professionals who challenge industry narratives may face personal and professional attacks, disciplinary actions, or reputational damage (Goldacre, 2013).

This tactic discourages open discussion about the benefits of generic, cost-effective treatments like metformin in preventive care, reinforcing the dominance of more expensive, proprietary medications in public health strategies.

Using Respected Publications to Publish Adverse Findings

Another method of influence is using respected, peer-reviewed journals to disseminate research that may skew against metformin use in preventive health. Industry-sponsored trials or observational studies can be designed to yield outcomes that favour newer, more profitable drugs over generics like metformin. By funding studies with carefully controlled parameters or by focusing on marginal risks, industry can ensure that adverse findings are emphasized in high-impact journals, creating fear or uncertainty about metformin's use in prevention.

These articles may receive extensive media coverage, especially if they are published in reputable journals or backed by respected researchers, further amplifying concerns about metformin. For example, studies that focus on rare cases of lactic acidosis in populations with severe kidney disease may be used to suggest that metformin is too dangerous for broader use, even though such risks are minimal in the general population. The media often simplifies and sensationalizes such findings, leading to public fear and professional caution (Lexchin, 2005).

Conclusion

While metformin has a well-established safety profile and considerable evidence supporting its use in preventing multiple chronic diseases, industry resistance to its widespread adoption as a preventive agent may manifest if Industry identifies this intervention as contrary to its financial interests. These include changing the narrative around metabolic dysfunction, publishing selective evidence, exaggerating risks, suppressing dissenting voices, and leveraging reputable journals to generate adverse findings.

As healthcare practitioners and policymakers consider the role of metformin in population-wide preventive health initiatives, it is crucial to recognize these industry tactics and ensure that evidence-based medicine, not financial incentives, drives public health strategies. While the TAME trial will provide more definitive evidence on metformin's role in aging, the current evidence strongly supports its use in high-risk populations. The challenge lies in overcoming the influence of industry to allow for cost-effective, generic interventions that could significantly reduce the burden of chronic disease worldwide.

© Dr. Christopher Maclay 2024

References

1. Inzucchi, S. E., et al. (2014). Management of hyperglycemia in type 2 diabetes: A patient-centered approach. *Diabetes Care*, 37(1), 14-80.
2. Michaels, D. (2008). *Doubt is Their Product: How Industry's Assault on Science Threatens Your Health*. Oxford University Press.
3. Smith, R. (2005). Medical journals are an extension of the marketing arm of pharmaceutical companies. *PLoS Medicine*, 2(5), e138.
4. Goldacre, B. (2013). *Bad Pharma: How Drug Companies Mislead Doctors and Harm Patients*. Faber & Faber.
5. Pollak, M. (2012). The effects of metformin on cancer prevention and therapy. *Nature Reviews Cancer*, 12(6), 448-460.
6. Lexchin, J. (2005). Impacts of direct-to-consumer advertising for prescription drugs. *Health Services Research*, 40(3), 981-997.

Chapter 11: A Comprehensive Risk-Benefit Analysis

As chronic diseases continue to escalate globally, particularly in older populations, the potential for pharmacological interventions such as metformin to mitigate this risk has become increasingly important. Metformin has gained recognition for its broader applications in chronic disease prevention. Based on both my 20 years of experience as a medical doctor and the current body of evidence, I believe metformin is an essential tool for individuals with significant risk factors for chronic disease. I also believe after age 40 those without significant risk for chronic disease are few are far between.

Don't ask me who is at risk, simply tell me who isn't?

For individuals with significant risk factors who have not achieved sufficient results with lifestyle changes, the benefits of metformin across these chronic disease domains cannot be overstated. In my opinion, it is a critical intervention for those who have tried and failed to reduce risk through non-pharmacological means. I also do not believe trials of Lifestyle Interventions need delay the use of metformin. They can be done simultaneously.

While the TAME trial (Targeting Aging with Metformin) plays out, there is compelling evidence to support the early use of metformin in these high-risk populations. This advice can then be adjusted. This chapter will summarise the data we have reviewed in earlier chapters, integrate a detailed risk-benefit analysis, highlight my clinical perspective, and expand on how metformin's potential benefits outweigh its risks.

RISK BENEFIT ANALYSIS

Here is a summary list based on the previous discussion regarding the use of metformin in preventing chronic disease and death:

1. Urgency of Intervention
- Rising rates of chronic diseases, diagnosed at increasingly younger ages, and a failure of current interventions to prevent this.
- Ageing populations, more diagnosis, more cost, more personal suffering.
- Explosion of risk factors; Obesity, Prediabetes and metabolic syndrome, age, PCOS, sedentarism, fatty liver, hypertension, dyslipidaemia etc

2. Current or Likely-to-be-Available Interventions
- Lifestyle advice interventions. Difficult adherence. Ignores the inherent characteristics of our modern society and environment responsible.
- Medications. Statins currently in use in high-risk populations, but with poor risk benefit ratio in low and normal risk groups, GLP-1 receptor agonists excessive cost, little long-term data.
- Emerging technologies: costly and little clinical data.

3. Likely Benefits of Using Metformin
- Delay or prevent the onset of chronic diseases: Diabetes, Dementia, Cancer, Cardiovascular disease, Chronic Kidney Disease.
- Reduction in mortality rates, increase in lifespan.
- Cost-effectiveness in high and low income nations.

4. Good side effect profile.

- Side effects: Gastrointestinal side effects, B12 deficiency, low risk of severe side effects. Easily monitored by a profession long versed in metformin use.

5. Pushback from Industry, if it occurs, may indicate the efficacy of this intervention.
- Pharmaceutical industry influence embedded in Medical Education, Medical regulators, Research Departments etc may view delaying chronic disease onset as a threat to financial interests. Anticipated responses would be Changing definitions of illness (e.g. metabolic dysfunction as a lifestyle issue), Exaggerating risks of metformin, Downplaying benefits, Delay guidelines including metformin, medical boards may punish practitioners who are early adopters, negative media coverage, rescheduling of medicines etc.

6. Summary Recommendations by Age Group
- Age 40 and over, no risk factors or disease. Offering Metformin. Individual risk assessment, likely to help, unlikely to harm. This is a clinically sound and reasonable option.

- Age 40 and over with risk factors: Aged over 50, elevated BMI, elevated waste circumference, PCOS, shift workers, high risk ethnicities, elevated fasting insulin or blood sugar level, elevated hsCRP, signs of fatty liver, abnormal blood lipids, hypertension, family history of chronic disease before age 60, sedentary lifestyle etc. This is the prime group for risk reduction. Patients should be recommended metformin as a preventative health option and monitored. Very likely to Help. Unlikely to harm.

- Age 40 and over with existing chronic disease (Diabetes, Cancer, Cardiovascular Disease, CKD or Neurocognitive Impairment).
  - Individuals aged 40 should be recommended metformin as dual primary and secondary prevention. Extremely likely to

benefit by slowing progressing of existing illness and delaying diagnosis of comorbidities. Unlikely to cause harm. Patients should be monitored.

Use at earlier ages should be considered if multiple risk factors are present.

Precautions:
Withhold is eGFR < 30.
Monitor for side effects. Cease if required.
Monitor B12 at least yearly, or simply supplement.
Adjust advice based on TAME trial update.

This summary can guide clinical decision-making and public health recommendations, ensuring appropriate use of metformin based on age, risk factors, and disease status.

Considering the Ethics of Widespread Metformin Use

1. Medicalization and Lifestyle Interventions

One of the key ethical concerns regarding the widespread use of metformin for prevention is the potential for overmedicalization—transforming normal aging into a medical condition requiring pharmaceutical intervention. I would direct readers to my book STOP AGEING to discuss why treating the ageing process specifically is the ideal way to prevent chronic disease and prolong lifespan. While metformin offers significant benefits, it is important not to downplay the importance of lifestyle interventions, which can prevent and manage many chronic diseases without the need for medications. In my experience, combining metformin with sustained lifestyle interventions offers the most effective preventive strategy.

2. Informed Consent and Autonomy

Informed consent is necessary in all medical interventions. This should not be suspended even in perceived 'emergencies' like the COVID19 Pandemic. In preventative health, including when considering metformin use in otherwise healthy individuals and those people with risk factors but no overt disease, informed consent is likewise crucial. Patients must be fully informed of the potential risks and benefits, and the decision to use metformin should respect their autonomy. I suggest the summary above could be used as a talking point.

3. Healthcare Costs and Accessibility: The affordability of metformin makes it an attractive option for large-scale disease prevention programs, particularly in low-resource settings. However, widespread use could also strain healthcare systems if individuals who are unlikely to benefit from metformin are prescribed the drug unnecessarily. Careful consideration must be given to the cost-effectiveness of prescribing metformin to different populations, ensuring that healthcare resources are allocated efficiently.

Conclusion

Metformin is, on balance and in my opinion, indicated for the prevention of chronic disease. It is a well-known, low cost, and safe intervention, with broad benefits across the most important diseases in the epidemic and a well understood mechanisms of action. Delays in implementation of this advice may result from pharmaceutical industry influence.

Lifestyle interventions and holistic preventative health plans are to be explored and implemented. I explore this in my book Anti Ageing Protocols.

I look forward to the publication of results from the TAME trial, which will provide further evidence on metformin's role. In the interim the risk benefit analysis is firmly in favour of use in people at risk of developing chronic disease. And who isn't?

References

1. Bannister, C.A., et al. "Can People with Type 2 Diabetes Live Longer than Those Without? A Comparison of Mortality in People Initiated with Metformin or Sulfonylurea Monotherapy and Matched, Non-Diabetic Controls." *Diabetes, Obesity and Metabolism*, 2014.
2. Barzilai, N., et al. "Metformin as a Tool to Target Aging." *Cell Metabolism*, 2016.
3. De Jager, J., et al. "Long Term Treatment with Metformin in Type 2 Diabetes and Vitamin B12 Deficiency." *Archives of Internal Medicine*, 2010.
4. Diabetes Prevention Program Research Group. "Reduction in the Incidence of Type 2 Diabetes with Lifestyle Intervention or Metformin." New England Journal of Medicine, 2002.
5. Imfeld, P., et al. "Metformin, Other Antidiabetic Drugs, and Risk of Alzheimer's Disease: A Population-Based Case-Control Study." Journal of the American Geriatrics Society, 2012.
6. Inzucchi, S.E., et al. "Management of Hyperglycemia in Type 2 Diabetes: A Patient-Centered Approach." Diabetes Care, 2014.
7. Pollak, M. "The Effects of Metformin on Cancer Prevention and Therapy." Nature Reviews Cancer, 2012.
8. Rhee, C.M., et al. "Metformin Use and Mortality in Patients with Advanced Chronic Kidney Disease." The Lancet, 2020.
9. UK Prospective Diabetes Study (UKPDS) Group. "Effect of Intensive Blood-Glucose Control with Metformin on

Complications in Overweight Patients with Type 2 Diabetes (UKPDS 34)." The Lancet, 1998.

Chapter 12: The TAME Trial

TAME Trial: Targeting Aging with MEtformin

I have mentioned the TAME trial repeatedly in prior chapters. The TAME (Targeting Aging with Metformin) trial, spearheaded by Dr. Nir Barzilai at the Albert Einstein College of Medicine, represents a groundbreaking effort to explore the use of metformin not merely for managing type 2 diabetes but as a potential tool to delay the onset of age-related diseases and extend healthspan. Unlike traditional studies that focus on treating specific illnesses, TAME seeks to investigate metformin's impact on the biology of aging itself, making it one of the first trials designed to treat aging as a modifiable risk factor for multiple chronic diseases.

Justification for the Trial

The rationale behind the TAME trial is based on accumulating evidence from both preclinical and clinical studies suggesting that metformin has significant effects on biological pathways associated with aging. Research has demonstrated that metformin can modulate processes such as insulin signalling, inflammation, mitochondrial function, and oxidative stress—key factors implicated in aging and chronic disease development (Barzilai et al., 2016).

By targeting these mechanisms, metformin could theoretically delay or prevent the onset of multiple age-related conditions, including cardiovascular disease, type 2 diabetes, cancer, chronic kidney disease, and neurodegenerative diseases like Alzheimer's. The trial aims to determine whether metformin can extend healthspan, which is the period of life free from disease, as well as lifespan.

Dr. Barzilai and his team have been strong advocates for redefining aging as a treatable condition, which could significantly shift the focus of healthcare from disease management to prevention. I strongly agree with this advocacy. The TAME trial represents the next step in advancing this new paradigm, and its findings could inform regulatory frameworks that consider aging as a modifiable risk factor for disease, opening the door to further pharmacological interventions aimed at extending healthy life.

Regulatory Reception

Convincing regulatory bodies, such as the U.S. Food and Drug Administration (FDA), to support the trial has been a challenge, primarily because ageing was not historically recognized as a "disease" in traditional medical frameworks. Metformin is already approved for the treatment of type 2 diabetes but demonstrating its efficacy as an "anti-aging" drug would require a shift in regulatory thinking.

The FDA typically approves drugs for specific disease treatments, and aging does not fall under that category. However, the TAME trial has sparked interest due to its potential to show that by delaying the onset of age-related diseases, the drug could be seen as targeting the underlying mechanisms of these conditions, rather than treating them individually. This approach could lead to a broader understanding of how to regulate and approve treatments that target the ageing processes (Campisi et al., 2019).

Study Design

The TAME trial is designed as a randomized, placebo-controlled study and aims to recruit approximately 3,000 adults aged 65-80 across 14 centres in the U.S. Participants will be followed over a period of six years to determine whether metformin can delay the development of age-related diseases. The diseases being tracked include cardiovascular disease, cancer, dementia, and stroke.

The trial design is unique in that its primary endpoint is not one single disease outcome, but rather a composite of several age-related diseases. This allows the researchers to observe whether metformin delays the onset of multiple conditions simultaneously, providing a more comprehensive picture of its effects on aging (Justice et al., 2018).

Key elements of the trial include:
- Duration: 6 years
- Participants: Approximately 3,000 older adults (ages 65-80)
- Primary Endpoint: Delay in the development of any major age-related disease (including cancer, cardiovascular events, dementia, and death)
- Design: Randomized, double-blind, placebo-controlled
- Secondary Outcomes: Healthspan measures, including cognitive function, physical performance, and quality of life.

Anticipated Results and Implications

The TAME trial is expected to provide preliminary results by the late 2020s. If successful, it could redefine the role of metformin in clinical practice, broadening its use from diabetes management to a key tool in delaying aging and preventing multiple chronic diseases. This could also lead to a shift in regulatory thinking, encouraging the approval of drugs that treat aging itself, rather than waiting for diseases to develop.

Should the TAME trial demonstrate (as is likely) that metformin can significantly delay the onset of major chronic diseases, it would likely pave the way for further research into other geroprotective drugs—compounds that can slow or reverse the aging process. Moreover, it could catalyse the development of new healthcare policies that focus on preventive medical care targeting the biological underpinnings of ageing as drivers for chronic disease.

Conclusion

The TAME trial represents a critical step in the evolution of preventive healthcare and anti-aging research. Led by Dr. Nir Barzilai, the study is designed to test whether metformin can delay the onset of multiple age-related diseases by targeting the biological mechanisms that drive aging. If successful, the TAME trial could usher in a new era of medicine, where ageing is treated as a modifiable risk factor, shifting the focus of healthcare from disease management to prevention and fundamentally reshaping the way we approach chronic disease and longevity.

References
1. Barzilai, N., et al. (2016). Metformin as a tool to target aging. *Cell Metabolism*, 23(6), 1060-1065.
2. Campisi, J., et al. (2019). From discoveries in ageing research to therapeutics for healthy ageing. *Nature*, 571(7764), 183-192.
3. Justice, J. N., et al. (2018). A geroscience perspective on immune aging and the TAME clinical trial. GeroScience, 40(3), 229-237.

Chapter 13: Beyond Metformin – The Future of Preventative Health

I do not foresee myself recommending Metformin for the prevention of Chronic Disease in 20 years' time. It could be the first large scale preventative health medicine, but certainly won't be the last. We will, and already do, have better interventions, although not at this price point, and not with this safety record – yet. Using metformin, as I suggest in this book, will introduce the concept of treating the underlying metabolic processes behind the development of diseases. This is desirable. And it will open a plethora of options.

As medical science continues to advance, the future of preventative health is becoming increasingly promising. The focus is shifting from merely managing diseases after they arise to proactively delaying their onset through innovative interventions and a holistic approach to healthcare. While metformin has emerged as a key player in this space, exciting new technologies and treatments are on the horizon, offering the potential to further extend healthspan, reduce chronic disease incidence, and ultimately improve the quality of life for millions.

Emerging Treatments and Interventions

Several emerging treatments and interventions hold the potential to revolutionize preventative health. While many of these are still in the early stages of research and development, they offer a glimpse of the future of medicine, where the focus is not only on treating diseases but preventing them at the root.

1. Senolytics: Senolytics are a class of drugs designed to selectively target and remove senescent cells—damaged cells

that no longer divide but contribute to inflammation and tissue dysfunction. These cells accumulate as we age and are thought to drive many of the chronic diseases associated with aging, such as cancer, cardiovascular disease, and neurodegeneration. Early studies in animals suggest that senolytics can improve healthspan by reducing inflammation and enhancing tissue repair, and clinical trials are now underway to test their effects in humans.

2. CRISPR and Gene Editing: CRISPR technology has revolutionized the field of genetics by allowing scientists to make precise edits to the genome. In the context of preventative health, CRISPR holds the potential to correct genetic mutations that predispose individuals to certain diseases, such as familial hypercholesterolemia, which increases the risk of heart disease. While this technology is still in its infancy in terms of widespread clinical application, the ability to correct disease-causing genes before symptoms arise could profoundly impact how we approach disease prevention in the future.

3. Personalized Medicine: The rise of personalized medicine, where treatments and preventive strategies are tailored to an individual's genetic makeup, lifestyle, and environment, is expected to play a significant role in the future of healthcare. Advances in genomics, proteomics, and metabolomics allow for more precise risk assessment and the development of targeted interventions. This means that in the future, preventative measures will not follow a "one-size-fits-all" approach but will be highly individualized, improving their effectiveness and minimizing risks.

4. Other Interventions: In addition to these cutting-edge technologies, other preventative treatments are also under investigation, including senomorphics, which aim to alter the behaviour of senescent cells without destroying them, and immunotherapies such as thymic regeneration, designed to

bolster the immune system's ability to prevent cancer and other age-related diseases.

While these emerging therapies hold great promise, they are a step beyond recommending Metformin, as many would consider them still largely in the research phase. They may not be widely available for many years. In the meantime, repurposing existing medications like metformin provides an immediate and cost-effective way to reduce the burden of chronic disease and promote healthy ageing, offering a bridge to these future innovations.

A Holistic Approach to Preventative Health

The future of preventative health will not rely on pharmaceuticals alone. To achieve the best outcomes, a holistic approach that combines lifestyle interventions with medications such as metformin is essential. Decades of research have shown that lifestyle factors such as diet, exercise, sleep, and circadian rhythm regulation are critical determinants of health. By integrating these factors into a comprehensive health plan, individuals can maximize the benefits of both lifestyle changes and pharmacological interventions.

1. Diet and Nutrition: A healthy diet rich in fruits, vegetables, whole grains, lean proteins, and healthy fats is a cornerstone of disease prevention. Numerous studies have shown that proper nutrition can reduce the risk of heart disease, diabetes, cancer, and neurodegenerative diseases. While metformin offers metabolic benefits, combining it with dietary interventions such as the Mediterranean or DASH diets can enhance its effects by optimizing blood sugar control, reducing inflammation, and improving cardiovascular health.

2. Physical Activity: Regular exercise is one of the most effective ways to prevent chronic diseases. It improves

cardiovascular health, enhances insulin sensitivity, reduces inflammation, and supports mental health. Combining physical activity with metformin may offer synergistic benefits, particularly in individuals at high risk for metabolic syndrome or diabetes. High-intensity interval training (HIIT) and strength training, in particular, have been shown to complement the effects of metformin on glucose regulation and metabolic health.

3. Circadian Rhythm and Sleep: Sleep quality and circadian rhythm regulation are increasingly recognized as vital components of health. Disrupted circadian rhythms and poor sleep are linked to a wide range of chronic diseases, including obesity, diabetes, cardiovascular disease, and cancer. Metformin has been shown to support circadian rhythm regulation, and when combined with strategies to improve sleep hygiene—such as maintaining a consistent sleep schedule, reducing exposure to artificial light at night, and managing stress—can further promote overall health and well-being.

4. Stress Management and Mental Health: Chronic stress and poor mental health are significant contributors to the development of chronic diseases. Techniques such as mindfulness, meditation, yoga, and cognitive-behavioural therapy can help reduce stress and improve mental health, potentially enhancing the benefits of metformin in reducing systemic inflammation and promoting healthy aging.

In the future, healthcare systems will need to embrace this integrative approach, combining evidence-based lifestyle modifications with pharmaceutical interventions like metformin to create comprehensive and personalized prevention plans. By focusing on the whole person rather than isolated disease states, it will be possible to prevent or delay the onset of chronic diseases, extending healthspan and improving quality of life.

Repurposing Medicines: Saving Suffering and Money Now

While the future of preventative health is bright, many of the emerging treatments will take years, if not decades, to be widely available. In the meantime, repurposing existing medications like metformin provides a valuable opportunity to save lives, reduce suffering, and alleviate the financial burden of chronic diseases.

1. Cost-Effectiveness of Metformin: As a generic drug, metformin is inexpensive and widely available, making it an ideal candidate for large-scale preventative health interventions. Compared to newer pharmaceuticals or cutting-edge technologies, metformin's low cost means it can be implemented in both high- and low-resource settings, providing an immediate solution to reducing chronic disease risk while the next generation of therapies is developed. The cost savings associated with reducing the incidence of diabetes, cardiovascular disease, cancer, and neurodegenerative diseases could be substantial, reducing the need for more expensive treatments and long-term care.

2. Immediate Impact on Public Health: The evidence supporting metformin's role in reducing the risk of multiple chronic diseases is robust. Studies have shown that metformin can lower the risk of cardiovascular disease, cancer, and neurodegenerative diseases, as well as delay the progression of type 2 diabetes. By implementing metformin as a preventive therapy now, healthcare systems can make an immediate impact on public health, reducing both morbidity and mortality while buying time for more advanced interventions like senolytics, CRISPR, and personalized medicine to reach clinical practice.

3. Gaining Time to Implement Future Preventive Health Measures: While waiting for future treatments to become

available, it is essential to optimize the use of existing tools like metformin. By leveraging metformin's broad-spectrum preventative effects, we can reduce the burden of chronic disease now and extend healthspan, allowing individuals to remain healthier for longer. This, in turn, provides the healthcare system with time to develop and implement more sophisticated preventive health measures as they become available.

Conclusion

The future of preventative health is exciting, with innovative treatments like senolytics, CRISPR, and personalised medicine on the horizon. However, these technologies are still years away from widespread availability. In the meantime, repurposing existing medications like metformin offers an immediate and cost-effective solution to reducing the risk of multiple chronic diseases and extending healthspan. By combining metformin with lifestyle interventions such as diet, exercise, and circadian rhythm regulation, we can create a comprehensive approach to health that not only addresses current challenges but also prepares us for the future of healthcare.

As we move forward, the focus should be on integrating these strategies into a holistic model of care that prioritises prevention, improves quality of life, and reduces the burden of chronic diseases worldwide.

References

1. Campisi, J., et al. "Senolytics: A Novel Approach to Target Aging and Age-Related Diseases." *Nature Reviews Drug Discovery*, 2020.

2. Jinek, M., et al. "A Programmable Dual-RNA-Guided DNA Endonuclease in Adaptive Bacterial Immunity." *Science*, 2012.

3. Personalized Medicine Coalition. "The Case for Personalized Medicine." *Journal of Personalized Medicine*, 2017.

4. Campbell, J.M., et al. "Metformin Reduces All-Cause Mortality and Diseases of Aging Independent of Its Effect on Diabetes Control: A Systematic Review and Meta-Analysis." *Ageing Research Reviews*, 2017.

5. Diabetes Prevention Program Research Group. "Reduction in the Incidence of Type 2 Diabetes with Lifestyle Intervention or Metformin." *New England Journal of Medicine*, 2002.

6. Barzilai, N., et al. "Metformin as a Tool to Target Aging." *Cell Metabolism*, 2016.

Conclusion

Metformin represents a transformative opportunity in the field of preventive healthcare. With a decades-long track record of safety, affordability, and efficacy, metformin has demonstrated its potential to reduce the risk of multiple chronic diseases, including type 2 diabetes, cardiovascular disease, chronic kidney disease, cancer, and neurodegenerative disorders. These conditions, driven by metabolic dysfunction, form the core of the chronic disease epidemic that is overwhelming healthcare systems globally.

The current approach to preventive health is largely reactive. It is focused on early detection, management of established illness, and lifestyle advice rather than true prevention. Despite well-meaning public health campaigns promoting diet, exercise, and lifestyle changes, the reality is that these efforts alone have not stemmed the rising tide of chronic disease. This is not a failure of individual willpower, but rather a failure of the healthcare system to address the underlying metabolic drivers of these diseases.

Metformin, by targeting core metabolic pathways, provides a direct intervention to reduce insulin resistance, inflammation, and oxidative stress—key contributors to these diseases. Its broad-spectrum benefits across multiple pathologies make it an ideal candidate for widespread preventive use, particularly in individuals with risk factors such as obesity, hyperinsulinemia, polycystic ovarian disease, age, impaired fasting glycemia, non-alcoholic steatohepatitis (NASH), hypertension, dyslipidaemia, and a significant family history of chronic illness... the list goes on.

While the TAME trial will provide further evidence on metformin's role in aging and chronic disease prevention, the available data already support its use in individuals at risk of developing chronic disease who have not achieved adequate risk reduction through lifestyle modifications alone. For consenting adults with clear risk factors, the potential benefits of using metformin far outweigh the risks, particularly when coupled with ongoing monitoring and lifestyle interventions.

A Vision for the Future

As we look to the future of healthcare, it is essential to adopt a proactive, prevention-first model. The evidence supporting metformin suggests that it could be a cornerstone in this paradigm shift. Its affordability and availability make it accessible for large-scale implementation, and its potential to delay or prevent the onset of chronic diseases could save millions in healthcare costs, reduce patient suffering, and extend healthy lifespan.

To achieve this vision, we must overcome systemic barriers—particularly those posed by industry influence, as discussed in earlier sections. The pharmaceutical industry may resist the broad adoption of metformin for preventive care due to financial motives, favouring more expensive and complex treatments that address diseases after they have already developed. However, the overwhelming evidence in support of metformin demands that we put public health first and act swiftly to integrate it into preventive health guidelines.

Call to Action

The need for an urgent shift toward prevention is clear. Policymakers, healthcare professionals, and public health advocates must come together to champion the use of metformin in preventive healthcare for those at risk of developing chronic diseases. The evidence is compelling, and the stakes are too high to wait for further validation while the chronic disease epidemic continues to worsen.

In conclusion, we must move toward a balanced, logical, and reasonable response—one that supports the use of metformin as a preventive intervention for consenting adults with risk factors for chronic disease. This is not about overmedicalizing the ageing process, but about providing individuals with the tools they need to extend their healthy years, reduce disease burden, and improve quality of life. The time for action is now, and metformin is a critical part of the solution.

EXTRAS

Thought Leaders

Further Reading

References

Thought Leaders

Thought leaders, with a focus on the prevention of chronic diseases and the potential use of interventions like metformin:

1. Dr. Nir Barzilai
   - Affiliation: Albert Einstein College of Medicine
   - Contributions: Dr. Barzilai is the principal investigator of the TAME trial and a leading voice advocating for using metformin to delay aging and prevent chronic diseases. His research focuses on understanding the genetic and metabolic mechanisms of aging, with a particular emphasis on using pharmacological interventions like metformin to prevent age-related conditions such as cardiovascular disease, cancer, and dementia.

2. Dr. James L. Kirkland
   - Affiliation: Mayo Clinic
   - Contributions: Dr. Kirkland is a pioneer in the study of senescence and its role in aging and chronic diseases. His work on senolytics, which target senescent cells, has significant implications for preventing chronic diseases like diabetes, cardiovascular disease, and kidney disease. His research intersects with metformin's potential to address cellular aging and reduce the burden of chronic illness.

3. Dr. João Pedro de Magalhães
   - Affiliation: University of Birmingham
   - Contributions: Dr. de Magalhães focuses on the genetic regulation of aging and how specific genes can be targeted to prevent chronic diseases. His work includes computational research to identify drugs that can modulate aging pathways, with metformin being a key candidate for preventing conditions such as cardiovascular disease and cancer by altering metabolic processes.

4. Dr. Judith Campisi
   - Affiliation: Buck Institute for Research on Aging
   - Contributions: Dr. Campisi's research on cellular senescence and inflammation explores how these processes contribute to chronic diseases such as cancer, cardiovascular disease, and neurodegeneration. Her work supports the use of interventions like metformin to mitigate inflammation and cellular damage, thereby preventing the onset of multiple chronic diseases.

5. Dr. Brian Kennedy
   - Affiliation: National University of Singapore
   - Contributions**: Dr. Kennedy has worked extensively on the biology of aging and how interventions like metformin can be used to delay the onset of chronic diseases. His research focuses on metabolic pathways and how targeting these pathways with pharmacological interventions could prevent diseases like diabetes, cardiovascular disease, and cancer, making him a key figure in translating aging research into clinical applications.

These thought leaders are driving the conversation around using interventions like metformin to prevent chronic diseases and extend healthspan. Their work is focused on finding practical solutions to reduce the burden of age-related diseases through metabolic and cellular interventions.

Further Reading

Here's a list of five relevant books that prioritize interventions to delay chronic disease and aging, including your own work:

1. STOP AGEING by Dr. Christopher Maclay (2024)
   - Overview: In Stop Ageing, Dr. Maclay advocates for the use of targeted interventions to delay the onset of chronic diseases by specifically targeting the ageing process. Drawing on his 20 years of experience in anti-aging and preventive medicine, the book advocates for a proactive, personalized approach to health, including the use of metformin and other therapies to enhance healthspan and prevent age-related diseases. Published independently in 2024, it serves as a comprehensive guide for individuals aiming to take control of their aging process.

2. Lifespan: Why We Age—and Why We Don't Have To by David A. Sinclair (2019)
   - Overview: In Lifespan, Dr. David Sinclair explores the science behind why we age and how interventions can potentially halt or reverse the aging process. He highlights key molecules like resveratrol and metformin, explaining how they interact with aging pathways such as sirtuins and mTOR. Sinclair argues for the potential to extend lifespan and healthspan by targeting the biological mechanisms of aging.

3. The End of Aging: The Quest to Halt the Biology of Time by David Stipp (2010)
   - Overview: This book focuses on the scientific breakthroughs that are changing the way we think about aging. Stipp explores how interventions like calorie restriction, gene therapy, and drugs like metformin could extend human lifespan by preventing chronic diseases. The End of Aging delves into the molecular biology of aging and the promising future of anti-aging interventions.

4. The Longevity Diet by Valter Longo (2018)
 - Overview: The Longevity Diet provides evidence-based strategies for extending healthspan and preventing chronic diseases through diet and fasting. Dr. Longo, a leading researcher in the field of aging, presents a dietary approach that mimics fasting, reducing inflammation and metabolic dysfunction, which are key drivers of chronic diseases. While the book focuses on nutrition, it complements pharmacological strategies like metformin in targeting the metabolic causes of aging.

5. The Longevity Economy: Unlocking the World's Fastest Growing, Most Misunderstood Market by Joseph F. Coughlin (2017)
 - Overview: Although not exclusively focused on medical interventions, The Longevity Economy discusses the economic implications of an aging population and the growing demand for anti-aging and preventive interventions. Coughlin addresses the future of aging and how innovations in medicine, including preventive strategies like metformin, will shape society's approach to health and aging.

These books provide a broad perspective on the science of aging and the interventions that could delay the onset of chronic diseases, each offering unique insights into how we can extend both healthspan and lifespan.

References

References cited and used in the preparation of this book have been listed at the end of the corresponding chapters.

Printed in Great Britain
by Amazon